Novel and Combination Therapies for Hepatitis C Virus

Editor

PAUL J. POCKROS

CLINICS IN LIVER DISEASE

www.liver.theclinics.com

Consulting Editor
NORMAN GITLIN

February 2013 • Volume 17 • Number 1

ELSEVIER

1600 John F. Kennedy Boulevard, Suite 1800 • Philadelphia, PA 19103-2899

http://www.theclinics.com

CLINICS IN LIVER DISEASE Volume 17, Number 1
February 2013 ISSN 1089-3261, ISBN-13: 978-1-4557-7112-7

Editor: Kerry Holland

Developmental Editor: Donald Mumford

Clinics in Liver Disease (ISSN 1089-3261) is published quarterly by Elsevier Inc., 360 Park Avenue South, New York, NY 10010-1710. Months of issue are February, May, August, and November. Business and Editorial Offices: 1600 John F. Kennedy Blvd., Ste. 1800, Philadelphia, PA 19103-2899. Customer Service Office: 3251 Riverport Lane, Maryland Heights, MO 63043. Periodicals postage paid at New York, NY and additional mailing offices. Subscription prices are $271.00 per year (U.S. individuals), $134.00 per year (U.S. student/resident), $365.00 per year (U.S. institutions), $360.00 per year (foreign individuals), $185.00 per year (foreign student/ resident), $440.00 per year (foreign institutions), $313.00 per year (Canadian individuals), $185.00 per year (Canadian student/resident), and $440.00 per year (Canadian institutions). Foreign air speed delivery is included in all *Clinics* subscription prices. All prices are subject to change without notice. **POSTMASTER:** Send address changes to *Clinics in Liver Disease*, Elsevier Health Sciences Division, Subscription Customer Service, 3251 Riverport Lane, Maryland Heights, MO 63043. **Customer Service: Telephone: 1-800-654-2452 (U.S. and Canada); 314-447-8871 (outside U.S. and Canada). Fax: 314-447-8029. E-mail: journalscustomer service-usa@elsevier.com (for print support); journalsonlinesupport-usa@elsevier.com (for online support).**

Reprints. For copies of 100 or more of articles in this publication, please contact the Commercial Reprints Department, Elsevier Inc., 360 Park Avenue South, New York, NY 10010-1710. Tel.: 212-633-3812; Fax: 212-462-1935; E-mail: reprints@elsevier.com.

Clinics in Liver Disease is covered in *MEDLINE/PubMed (Index Medicus)*, Science Citation Index Expanded, Journal Citation Reports/Science Edition, and Current Contents/Clinical Medicine.

Printed and bound by CPI Group (UK) Ltd, Croydon, CR0 4YY

Transferred to digital print 2012

Contributors

CONSULTING EDITOR

NORMAN GITLIN, MD, FRCP (LONDON), FRCPE (EDINBURGH), FACG, FACP
Formerly, Professor of Medicine, Chief of Hepatology, Emory University; Currently, Consultant, Atlanta Gastroenterology Associates, Atlanta, Georgia

GUEST EDITOR

PAUL J. POCKROS, MD
Head, Division of Gastroenterology and Hepatology, Director of Liver Disease Center and SC Liver Research Consortium, Scripps Clinic and Clinical Director of Research, Scripps Translational Science Institute, La Jolla, California

AUTHORS

JAMES R. BURTON JR, MD
Associate Professor of Medicine, Medical Director of Liver Transplantation, Department of Medicine, University of Colorado Denver, Aurora, Colorado

ANUSHREE CHATTERJEE, PhD
Theoretical Biology and Biophysics; Center for Nonlinear Studies, Los Alamos National Laboratory, Los Alamos, New Mexico

DOUGLAS T. DIETERICH, MD
Professor of Medicine, Division of Liver Diseases, Department of Medicine, Mount Sinai School of Medicine, New York, New York

JENNIFER C. ESPINALES
Department of Biological Sciences, University of Texas at Brownsville, Brownsville, Texas

GREGORY T. EVERSON, MD
Professor of Medicine, Director of Hepatology, Department of Medicine, University of Colorado Denver, Aurora, Colorado

IRA M. JACOBSON, MD
Professor of Medicine, Chief, Division of Gastroenterology and Hepatology, Director, Center for Study of Hepatitis C, New York-Presbyterian Hospital/Weill Cornell Medical College, New York, New York

ARUN B. JESUDIAN, MD
Gastroenterology Fellow, Division of Gastroenterology and Hepatology, New York-Presbyterian Hospital/Weill Cornell Medical College, New York, New York

PAUL Y. KWO, MD
Professor of Medicine, Medical Director, Liver Transplantation, Gastroenterology/Hepatology Division, Indiana University School of Medicine, Indianapolis, Indiana

ERIC J. LAWITZ, MD, AGAF, CPI
Alamo Medical Research, San Antonio, Texas

ANNA SUK-FONG LOK, MD
Professor of Medicine, Division of Gastroenterology and Hepatology, University of Michigan Health System, University of Michigan, Ann Arbor, Michigan

VALÉRIE MARTEL-LAFERRIÈRE, MD
Fellow, Division of Liver Diseases, Department of Medicine, Mount Sinai School of Medicine, New York, New York

FERNANDO E. MEMBRENO, MD, MSc
Alamo Medical Research, San Antonio, Texas

ALAN S. PERELSON, PhD
Theoretical Biology and Biophysics, Los Alamos National Laboratory, Los Alamos, New Mexico

PAUL J. POCKROS, MD
Head, Division of Gastroenterology and Hepatology, Director of Liver Disease Center and SC Liver Research Consortium, Scripps Clinic and Clinical Director of Research, Scripps Translational Science Institute, La Jolla, California

PATRICK F. SMITH, PhD
Clinical Pharmacology, Pharma Research and Early Development, Roche, Nutley, New Jersey

JOHN M. VIERLING, MD, FACP
Professor of Medicine and Surgery, Chief of Hepatology, Director of Baylor Liver Health, Director of Advanced Liver Therapies, St. Luke's Episcopal Hospital, Baylor College of Medicine, Houston, Texas

JOHN W. WARD, MD
Division of Viral Hepatitis, Centers for Disease Control and Prevention, Atlanta, Georgia

Contents

Hepatitis C virus (HCV) is the most common blood-borne infection in the United States. HCV infection is a leading cause of chronic liver disease, end-stage liver disease, and liver transplantation. Newly available therapies can clear HCV in most infected persons who receive treatment. However, many persons living with HCV infection are unaware of their infection status, including those born during 1945–1965 (a population at increased risk for chronic hepatitis C in the United States). This review highlights the epidemiology of hepatitis C and the importance of HCV testing and linkage to care in an era of more effective antiviral therapies.

Mathematical modeling of hepatitis C viral kinetics has been an important tool in understanding hepatitis C virus (HCV) infection dynamics and in estimating crucial in vivo parameters characterizing the effectiveness of HCV therapy. Because of the introduction of direct-acting antiviral agents, there is a need to extend previous models so as to understand, characterize, and compare various new HCV treatment regimens. Here we review recent modeling efforts in this direction.

In the direct-acting antiviral (DAA) era of hepatitis C virus (HCV) therapy, health care providers must be knowledgeable about genotype and subtype of HCV infection and interpretation of quantitative HCV viral assays to monitor treatment responses. They may also choose to assess interleukin 28B genotypes or resistance-associated variants after ineffective DAA therapy. DAA therapies require understanding of performance characteristics of quantitative HCV RNA assays and the definitions of terms used to report results. Only quantitative HCV RNA assays with a limit of detection of 10 to 15 IU/mL are appropriate for managing patients on DAA therapy.

Telaprevir is a recently approved direct-acting antiviral against hepatitis C virus (HCV) that works through inhibition of the NS3/4A serine protease inhibitor. Phase 2b and 3 studies have shown marked increase in sustained virologic response rates in both treatment-naïve and treatment-experienced patients with HCV genotype 1 treated with a telaprevir-containing regimen compared with pegylated interferon (Peg-IFN) and ribavirin alone. The most commonly observed side effects of telaprevir therapy are anemia to a greater degree than that observed with Peg-IFN/ribavirin alone; eczematous rash, which can be severe in a minority of patients; and anorectal discomfort.

The addition of boceprevir to peginterferon and ribavirin has improved sustained response rates markedly. Boceprevir is effective in treatment naïve, relapsers, partial responders, and null responders. Those with advanced fibrosis require 44 weeks of boceprevir therapy after a 4-week peg/ribavirin lead-in. The main side effect with boceprevir is anemia and ribavirin dose reduction is an effective strategy. This review examines the current treatment paradigm of boceprevir-based treatment of chronic hepatitis C, examining treatment paradigms, predictors of response, futility rules, as well as preliminary results from studies examining boceprevir efficacy in additional populations. Further follow-up in these cohorts will be required.

More than one-third of listed potential liver recipients in the US are infected with the hepatitis C virus (HCV). Recurrence of infection with HCV after liver transplantation is associated with accelerated graft loss and diminished patient survival. Current HCV treatments using peginterferon and ribavirin either alone or with first generation protease inhibitors (telaprevir, boceprevir) are limited by suboptimal viral response, drug-drug interaction, and side effects, some of which may be graft- or life-threatening. Rapid advances in new drug therapy for HCV promise to improve outcomes, reduce side effects and drug-drug interaction, shorten treatment duration, and simplify treatment regimens.

Monotherapy is an ineffective way to treat hepatitis C and it leads to rapid development of resistance. An increasing number of drugs are currently being developed for the treatment of hepatitis C. This allows combination strategies that can overcome the development of resistance and improve sustained virologic response rates. This article focuses on the 2 main strategies in development: quadruple combination therapies, including pegylated-interferon and triple/quadruple pegylated-interferon free combination therapies. If the first combinations are leading to extremely high sustained virologic responses, the second ones offer hope that the era of pegylated-interferon will end soon.

Nucleoside/nucleotide analogue polymerase inhibitors (NPIs) are analogues of natural substrates that bind the active site of NS5B and terminate viral RNA chain generation and generally provide a high genetic barrier to resistance and are effective in all genotypes. NPIs such as sofosbuvir (GS-7977) show high antiviral activities that, together with their high genetic barrier to resistance, suggest that they are optimal backbone candidates for all-oral combination therapies. Several trials are ongoing to further define the potential of all-oral regimens with sofosbuvir (GS-7977). Recent interim analyses indicate that many patients treated with only 2 direct-acting antiviral agents experience viral breakthrough, which can be significantly reduced by the addition of ribavirin without pegylated interferon α.

NS5A protein plays a key role in hepatitis C virus (HCV) replication. Daclatasvir (DCV, BMS-790052) is a first-in-class inhibitor of the HCV NS5A replication complex with potent antiviral activity but a low barrier to resistance. DCV as triple therapy in combination with pegylated interferon and ribavirin resulted in a high rate of early virologic response in treatment-naïve patients with genotype 1 infection; as quadruple therapy in combination with asunaprevir (BMS-650032, NS3 protease inhibitor), pegylated interferon, and ribavirin, it resulted in a high rate of sustained virologic response in genotype 1 prior null responders.

Non-nucleoside polymerase inhibitors have several limitations including low to moderate potency, a low barrier to resistance, unlikely to cross genotype activity, genotype potency 1b > 1a, and hyperbilirubinemia for 2 of the drugs (tegobuvir and BI-207127). These drugs will have no role in monotherapy and may have only a limited role in triple therapy. They could be part of a quadruple therapy regimen or a triple or quadruple interferon-free regimen. Several issues remain unclear at the time of this review; the role of these compounds including minimal dosing required, safety, and cost remains to be clarified.

This article highlights a unique time in the history of Hepatitis C therapy. In the last few years new families of direct-acting antivirals have emerged, that block different viral proteins to interrupt viral replication, such as protease, NS5A inhibitors, and NS5B inhibitors. There are few host-targeted agents in development; currently cyclophilin inhibitors are the only host-targeted agents in advanced development. One of these new agents has now progressed to phase 3 clinical trials; in this review article their potential role as a future therapy to cure Hepatitis C is discussed.

CLINICS IN LIVER DISEASE

NOW AVAILABLE FOR YOUR iPhone and iPad

Preface

Novel and Combination Therapies for Hepatitis C Virus

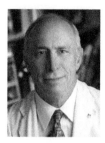

Paul J. Pockros, MD
Guest Editor

Tremendous progress has been made toward the development of interferon-free hepatitis C therapy in the years since I last edited this topic for *Clinics in Liver Disease* in 2009. Since that time, a number of therapies have been shown to work in a whole range of different combinations and treatment schedules. It is clear now that interferon-free regimens are a realistic scenario for the upcoming years. However, there remain a number of significant challenges to overcome. Most of the difficult-to-treat patient populations, including patients with cirrhosis, previous interferon null-responders, HIV/hepatitis C virus (HCV) coinfected and decompensated patients, and those with posttransplant HCV infection, have not yet been studied.

Further, we have seen that a number of interferon-free combinations have efficacy limitations in certain viral subtypes or IL28B genotypes. There are a number of questions regarding drug interactions, side effects, and treatment durations that have not yet been answered. There are also some nagging concerns about antiviral drug resistance, late viral relapse, and, last of all, the cost of these regimens. These issues have recently become more pressing in the United States because of the institution of birth-cohort screening of all individuals born between 1945 and 1965. This represents roughly one-third of the US population and will ultimately identify a huge group of

Clin Liver Dis 17 (2013) xi–xii
http://dx.doi.org/10.1016/j.cld.2012.09.012
1089-3261/13/$ – see front matter © 2013 Elsevier Inc. All rights reserved.

liver.theclinics.com

patients with chronic HCV who require treatment. We attempt to address each of these issues and concerns in the following articles.

Paul J. Pockros, MD
Division of Gastroenterology and Hepatology
Scripps Clinic and Scripps Translational Science Institute
10666 North Torrey Pines Road
La Jolla, CA 92037, USA

E-mail address:
pockros.paul@scrippshealth.org

The Epidemiology of Chronic Hepatitis C and One-Time Hepatitis C Virus Testing of Persons Born During 1945 to 1965 in the United States

John W. Ward, MD

KEYWORDS

- Hepatitis C virus • HCV testing • Baby boomers • HCV testing recommendations

KEY POINTS

- Despite overall declines in hepatitis C incidence, hepatitis C virus (HCV) continues to be transmitted; new infections are increasing in some populations, including young persons who inject drugs.
- As indicated by a national health survey, an estimated 3.2 million persons are living with HCV in the United States.
- Chronic hepatitis C is a major cause of liver disease, including hepatocellular carcinoma, the fastest growing cancer-related cause of death.
- Many if not most persons living with viral hepatitis remain undiagnosed.
- To realize the health benefits anticipated from new HCV therapies, approaches to testing must be strengthened and updated as HCV epidemiology evolves, more persons must become aware of their HCV infection status through 1-time HCV testing, and those found infected must be linked to care and treatment.
- The Centers for Disease Control and Prevention recommendation for a 1-time HCV test for persons born during 1945 to 1965 is a cost-effective approach to reducing HCV-associated morbidity and mortality.
- Successful implementation of this policy requires public health, clinical care providers, laboratories, and third-party payers to work together to improve HCV testing, care, and treatment in the United States.

INTRODUCTION

Hepatitis C virus (HCV) is the most common blood-borne infection in the United States. An estimated 4.1 million persons are infected with HCV, of whom 3.2 (2.7–3.9) million have chronic infection.[1] HCV is most often transmitted among persons who inject drugs

Division of Viral Hepatitis, Centers for Disease Control and Prevention, 1600 Clifton Road, NE, Atlanta, GA 30333, MS G-37, USA
E-mail address: jww4@cdc.gov

Clin Liver Dis 17 (2013) 1–11
http://dx.doi.org/10.1016/j.cld.2012.09.011
1089-3261/13/$ – see front matter Published by Elsevier Inc.

(PWID) and through exposures to HCV-contaminated blood and blood products in health care settings with inadequate infection control. Sexual contact and perinatal exposures also serve as modes of transmission. Once infected with HCV, 75% to 85% of persons remain chronically infected.[2] Chronic infection with HCV can result in liver inflammation, cirrhosis, and liver cancer; HCV infection is a leading cause of chronic liver disease, end-stage liver disease, and eventual need for liver transplantation. HCV-associated mortality is increasing in the United States, recently surpassing the number of deaths attributed to human immunodeficiency virus (HIV)/AIDS (**Fig. 1**).[3] Newly available therapies can clear HCV (ie, achieve virologic cure) in most HCV-infected persons who receive treatment, and numerous additional treatments undergoing clinical trials show promise for further benefits.[4–6] However, many persons living with HCV infection are unaware of their infection status.[7–12] This review highlights the epidemiology of hepatitis C and the priorities for prevention of HCV transmission and disease in an era of more effective antiviral therapies.

HCV TRANSMISSION

Approximately 60% to 70% of HCV-infected persons are asymptomatic during the acute phase of infection. The average time from viral exposure to a positive antibody to HCV (anti-HCV) seroconversion is 8 to 9 weeks, and anti-HCV can be detected in more than 97% of persons by 6 months after exposure.[13–15] The most efficient route of HCV transmission is parenteral exposure to blood, including transfusions and injections. Among PWID, HCV infection is acquired rapidly after initiation of injecting, and incidence rates of HCV infection are highest among young PWID.[16–19] Risks for HCV infection among PWID include years of injection drug use, injection frequency, sharing practices, and sex work; HCV infection prevalence is strongly associated with duration of injection drug use, reaching 65% to 90% among long-term injectors.[16,18] High rates of HCV among PWID largely explain the high rates among incarcerated populations.[20]

Health care-associated exposures also are major sources of HCV transmission, including receipt of blood not screened for HCV, unsafe injections, and other health care procedures. In the United States, reports of nosocomial HCV transmission have increased in recent years. From 1998 to 2012, the Centers for Disease Control and Prevention (CDC) investigated at least 33 outbreaks of HCV infection linked to

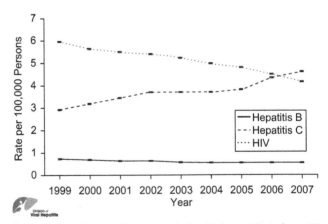

Fig. 1. Age-adjusted rates of mortality associated with hepatitis B, hepatitis C, and HIV, United States, 1999 to 2007. (*Data from* Centers for Disease Control. Sentinel counties study of viral hepatitis and state disease surveillance.)

transmission in variety of care settings (CDC unpublished data, 2012).[21] The risk of HCV transmission after a needlestick exposure to blood from a source positive for anti-HCV is 1.8% (range: 0%–7%).[22–25] Generally, HCV is less efficiently transmitted by mucosal exposures to blood, although noninjection-drug users who sniff cocaine and other drugs have increased risks for HCV infection.[26] HCV in plasma can survive drying and environmental exposure to room temperature for at least 16 hours, supporting epidemiologic studies that implicate injection equipment, household exposures, and unsafe barbering practices as modes of HCV transmission.[27]

HCV also can be transmitted through perinatal and sexual exposures. The risk of perinatal transmission is 4% to 5% for infants born to HCV-infected, HIV-negative women, increasing to 17% to 25% among infants born to women coinfected with HCV and HIV.[28,29] Although sexual transmission of HCV is not as common as other transmission modes, case-control studies have reported an association between acquiring hepatitis C and exposure to an HCV-infected sex contact or exposure to multiple sex partners.[30] In addition, 15% to 20% of newly infected patients report a history of sexual exposures in the absence of percutaneous risk factors for HCV.[31] Risk of HCV transmission by sexual exposure varies by population. HCV prevalence is low (1.5%) among long-term heterosexual partners of persons with chronic HCV infection.[32–35] In contrast, coinfection with HIV-1 seems to increase the risk of HCV sexual transmission among men who have sex with men (MSM). In the last several years, outbreaks of HCV infection have been reported among HIV-infected MSM without a history of injection drug use in Europe and more recently, the United States.[36–39]

HEPATITIS C INCIDENCE

Hepatitis C incidence in the United States peaked at approximately 240,000 new infections per year in the early to mid-1980s, before the discovery of HCV in 1988 (**Fig. 2**).[40,41] In the following years, incidence of hepatitis C declined steadily until 2004, when incidence leveled at an estimated 15,000 to 20,000 new infections (0.3 cases per 100,000 population). In 2010, an estimated 17,000 new HCV infections occurred, with injection drug use being the most commonly reported risk factor.[42] However, the number of new HCV infections seems to be increasing in some areas of the United States. For example, from 2002 to 2009, Massachusetts observed an increase in reports of HCV among persons 15 to 24 years of age.[43] These cases

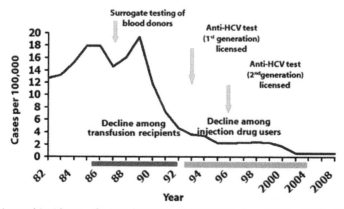

Fig. 2. Estimated incidence of acute hepatitis C: United States, 1982 to 2009. (*Courtesy of* Sentinel Counties Study of Viral Hepatitis and State Disease Surveillance; with permission.)

were reported from all areas of the state; injection drug use was the most common risk for HCV transmission. Other states have reported similar increases.[44] Taken together, these data suggest a new wave of HCV transmission among populations of adolescents and young adults who have recently begun to inject drugs.

HEPATITIS C PREVALENCE

Based on a national health survey, an estimated 3.2 (2.7–3.9) million persons are living with HCV in the United States.[1] However, because this survey excludes or underestimates populations at greatest risk for hepatitis C (eg, incarcerated persons), an additional 500,000 to 1,000,000 persons are likely infected with HCV.[45] Chronic hepatitis C is a major cause of liver disease; approximately 36% of all persons awaiting liver transplant and at least 50% of all persons with hepatocellular carcinoma (HCC) are HCV-infected.[46,47] With a 2.5% annual increase, HCC-associated deaths are increasing faster than other causes of cancer deaths.[48]

Both acute and chronic HCV infections are relatively asymptomatic. Therefore, persons living with HCV are often unaware that they are infected until late in the course of disease, typically resulting in a decades-long latency between acquisition of HCV and the development of end-stage liver disease and death. After 30 years of infection, persons living with HCV have a 15% to 35% and 1% to 3% risk for cirrhosis and HCC, respectively.[49,50] However, the risk for disease progression continues over a lifetime, and risks of HCV-related morbidity and mortality are expected to increase as persons with chronic hepatitis C grow older. During the next 40 to 50 years, a projected 1.76 million persons with untreated HCV infection are expected to develop cirrhosis, with a peak prevalence of 1 million cases occurring from the mid-2020s to the mid-2030s; approximately 400,000 will develop HCC.[51] Of persons with hepatitis C who do not receive needed care and treatment, approximately 1 million are expected to die from HCV-related complications.

HCV INFECTION PREVALENCE AMONG PERSONS BORN DURING 1945 TO 1965

Of persons living with hepatitis C, an estimated 76% are adults born during 1945 to 1965 (a population known as baby boomers in the United States).[52] As this population likely has been infected for several decades, HCV-associated morbidity and mortality are on the increase. Hepatitis C-associated mortality increased 50% during 1999 to 2007 (annual mortality change: +0.18 deaths per 100,000 population per year). In 2007, HCV caused 15,106 deaths, 73.4% of which occurred among persons aged 45 to 64 years (roughly corresponding to the baby boomer cohort); the median age of death was 57 years, approximately 20 years less than the average life span of persons living in the United States.[3] A study of HCV-infected military veterans in care from 1996 to 2003, many of whom were born during 1945 to 1965, reported increased rates of cirrhosis (50%) and HCC (20-fold) during the study period.[53]

ECONOMIC IMPLICATIONS OF HCV INFECTION

HCV infection poses an economic burden in the United States, resulting in lost productivity and additional health care costs for infected persons. Compared with other employees, those with HCV infection require more sick leave per year and short-term and long-term disability, resulting in more absences from work and lost productivity.[54] HCV infection also results in substantial direct costs for medical care. A study of medical reimbursement claims from 2002 to 2006 revealed that hospitalization occurred in 24% of HCV-infected patients compared with 7% of controls.[55]

Annual health care costs for HCV-infected persons were 5-fold higher than those for other patients, totaling $20,961 and exceeding costs for other common diseases, including cardiovascular diseases ($18,965) and diabetes mellitus ($9677). Numerous studies reveal the cost-effective benefits of HCV screening and care for populations at risk for hepatitis C[56,57]; In 1 study, HCV therapy followed by viral clearance reduced annual costs of patient care by half.[55]

NEW TREATMENTS FOR HCV

Therapy can clear HCV infection from the body, resulting in sustained virologic response (SVR), which indicates virologic cure. Until 2011, approximately 40% of patients who completed a 48-week course of a standard therapeutic regimen of pegylated interferon and ribavirin achieved SVR.[2] In 2011, 2 new agents, boceprevir and telaprevir, were licensed for treatment of HCV, representing the first direct-acting agents (DAAs) with specific activity against HCV infection. Compared with pegylated interferon/ribavirin therapy alone, the addition of telaprevir or boceprevir to this regimen increases SVR rates from 38% to 63% and 44% to 75%, respectively.[4,5] Guided by patients' HCV RNA level during therapy, the course of treatment can be as short as 24 to 28 weeks for patients with optimal viral response. However, serious adverse events during therapy continue to affect 5% to 10% of patients.[2] Approximately 20 HCV treatments (eg, protease and polymerase inhibitors) are undergoing phase II or phase III clinical trials.[6] These agents are expected to decrease adverse events, shorten the duration of therapy, and improve treatment effectiveness; they also may lead to an all-oral regimen for HCV treatment, without the need for pegylated interferon.[58] Treatment recommendations will change as new medications become available for use in the United States.[59]

TESTING AND LINKAGE TO CARE

Only through HCV testing with linkage to care can HCV-infected persons receive needed clinical management and treatment. However, at a time of increasing HCV-related morbidity and mortality, hepatitis C is an underrecognized and undertreated disease. In 2007, fewer than 85,000 persons were treated for HCV infection (a fraction of the estimated 3.2 million persons infected with the virus).[11] Some patients do not meet the recommended criteria to receive therapy, and others have conditions (eg, depression) for which therapy is contraindicated.[2,59] However, as reported by the Institute of Medicine, other barriers to improved health outcomes for persons living with hepatitis C exist, including the lack of awareness of HCV infection as a health threat by policy makers and the public; inadequate numbers of clinicians trained to test, manage, and treat HCV-infected patients; and the low percentage of persons aware of their infection.[60]

Since 1998, CDC has recommended HCV testing for certain high-risk populations, including persons who have ever injected illegal drugs; recipients of transfusions and transplants before 1992; patients with selected medical conditions (eg, dialysis and increased alanine transaminase level); health care and public safety workers after needlesticks, sharps, or mucosal exposures to HCV-positive blood; and children born to HCV-positive women.[61] However, strategies based on risk ascertainment and certain medical indications have been implemented with variable success. Of participants in the National Health and Nutrition Examination Survey, only 3 (7%) of 46 HCV-infected persons reported having been tested based on known HCV-related risk factors.[12] Of HCV-infected persons, only 45% to 85% have been tested for HCV[7-9,11,12]; these low rates reflect the challenges faced by clinicians and patients when discussing sensitive personal behaviors, particularly when they are not relevant to the current medical care visit.

To overcome barriers to risk-based approaches to HCV testing, CDC considered alternative public health strategies. Because persons born during 1945 to 1965 have a 5-fold greater prevalence of HCV infection (3.25%) than other adults (**Fig. 3**), accounting for more than three-fourths (76.5%) of the total anti-HCV prevalence and 73% of HCV-related mortality in the United States, CDC is now recommending HCV testing of persons born during these years.[62] In addition to testing adults of all ages at high risk for HCV infection, CDC recommends that adults born during 1945 to 1965 should receive 1-time testing for HCV without previous ascertainment of HCV risk (**Box 1**). Further, all persons identified with HCV infection should receive a brief alcohol screening and intervention as clinically indicated, followed by referral to appropriate care and treatment services for HCV infection and related conditions. With full implementation of this strategy, CDC estimates that 800,000 persons currently unaware of their HCV infection will be identified; more than 120,000 HCV-related deaths will be averted if these persons are linked to appropriate care and DAA treatment.[63]

Critical to the effectiveness of CDC's recommendation for 1-time HCV testing among persons born during 1945 to 1965 is consistent implementation by the clinicians serving persons in this birth cohort and an understanding of the need for HCV testing by the targeted population. Guided by a US Department of Health and Human Services (HHS) action plan for viral hepatitis that outlines explicit steps to improve coordination across HHS agencies,[64] CDC has initiated several activities to foster implementation of the new HCV testing recommendations. To improve awareness of viral hepatitis among the public and providers, CDC recently launched the *Know More Hepatitis* multimedia campaign (http://www.cdc.gov/knowmorehepatitis), which provides persons born during 1945 to 1965 with targeted HCV testing messages and a risk-assessment tool. The campaign also provides public health and clinical care providers online training opportunities. To increase capacity for HCV testing and linkage to care in fiscal year 2012, CDC provided funds to support HCV testing and linkage to care in diverse clinical settings. Further, funds were allocated to replicate models of case-based learning to help primary care providers deliver high-quality HCV-related care and treatment comparable with that provided by medical specialists.[65]

Several mechanisms are in place for the collection of surveillance and epidemiologic data to evaluate trends in HCV testing, care, and treatment. For example, data on

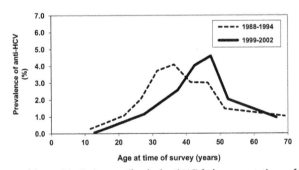

Fig. 3. Prevalence of hepatitis C virus antibody (anti-HCV), by age at time of survey — Third National Health and Nutrition Examination Survey (NHANES III) 1988–1994 and NHANES IV, 1999–2002. (*Data from* Armstrong GL, Wasley A, Simard EP, et al. The prevalence of hepatitis C virus infection in the United States, 1999 through 2002. Ann Intern Med 2006;144(10):705–14.)

Box 1
CDC recommendation for 1-time HCV testing persons born during 1945 to 1965

- In addition to testing adults at risk for HCV infection, CDC recommends that:
  - Adults born during 1945 to 1965 should receive 1-time testing for HCV without previous ascertainment of HCV risk factor. (Strong recommendation, moderate quality of evidence.)
  - All persons with identified HCV infection should receive a brief alcohol screening and intervention as appropriate, followed by referral to appropriate care and treatment services for HCV infection and related conditions as indicated. (Strong recommendation, moderate quality of evidence.)

---

acute and chronic HCV infection are reported to CDC through state/local hepatitis C surveillance systems. To evaluate clinical management, CDC, in collaboration with the CDC Foundation's Viral Hepatitis Action Coalition, is monitoring the quality and impact of care and treatment of more than 10,000 HCV-infected patients. In the future, questions regarding HCV testing will be incorporated into national health surveys to help assess the impact of HCV testing recommendations, and data compiled from outpatient and inpatient health records will be analyzed to detect changes in HCV testing patterns. CDC also evaluates point of care and other technologies to facilitate HCV testing and surveillance.[66]

SUMMARY

Despite overall declines in hepatitis C incidence, HCV continues to be transmitted; new infections are increasing in some populations, including young PWID. Chronic HCV infections acquired in decades past are now manifesting, damaging the liver and leading to increases in HCV-related morbidity and mortality; hepatitis C represents a major health disparity for persons born during 1945 to 1965. Many if not most persons living with viral hepatitis remain undiagnosed. To realize the health benefits anticipated from new HCV therapies, approaches to testing must be strengthened and updated as HCV epidemiology evolves, more persons must become aware of their HCV infection status through 1-time HCV testing, and those found infected must be linked to care and treatment. The CDC recommendation for a 1-time HCV test for persons born during 1945 to 1965 is a cost-effective approach to reducing HCV-associated morbidity and mortality.[63] Successful implementation of this policy requires public health, clinical care providers, laboratories, and third-party payers to work together to improve HCV testing, care, and treatment in the United States.

REFERENCES

1. Armstrong GL, Wasley A, Simard EP, et al. The prevalence of hepatitis C virus infection in the United States, 1999 through 2002. Ann Intern Med 2006;144: 705–14.
2. Ghany MG, Strader DB, Thomas DL, et al. Diagnosis, management, and treatment of hepatitis C: an update [Practice Guideline]. Hepatology 2009;49: 1335–74.
3. Ly K, Xing J, Klevens M, et al. The growing burden of mortality from viral hepatitis in the US, 1999–2007. Ann Intern Med 2012;156(4):271.
4. Jacobson I, McHutchison J, Dusheiko G, et al. Telaprevir for previously untreated chronic hepatitis C virus infection. N Engl J Med 2011;364(25):2405–16.

5. Poordad F, McCone J, Bacon B, et al. Boceprevir for untreated chronic HCV genotype 1 infection. N Engl J Med 2011;364(13):1195–206.
6. Asselah T, Marcellin P. Direct acting antivirals for the treatment of chronic hepatitis C: one pill a day for tomorrow. Liver Int 2012;32(Suppl 1):S88–102.
7. Roblin DW, Smith BD, Weinbaum CM, et al. Hepatitis C virus screening practices and prevalence in a managed care organization. Am J Manag Care 2011;17: 548–55.
8. Southern WN, Drainoni ML, Smith BD, et al. Hepatitis C testing practices and prevalence in a high-risk urban ambulatory care setting. J Viral Hepat 2011;18: 474–81.
9. Spradling PR, Rupp L, Moorman AC, et al. Hepatitis B and C virus infection among 1.2 million persons with access to care: factors associated with testing and infection prevalence. Clin Infect Dis 2012;55(8):1047–55.
10. Moorman AC, Gordon SC, Rupp LB, et al. Baseline characteristics and mortality among people in care for chronic viral hepatitis: the Chronic Hepatitis Cohort Study (CHeCS). Clin Infect Dis 2012. [Epub ahead of print].
11. Volk ML, Tocco R, Saini S, et al. Public health impact of antiviral therapy for hepatitis C in the United States. Hepatology 2009;50:1750–5.
12. Denniston MM, Klevens RM, McQuillan GM, et al. Awareness of infection, knowledge of hepatitis C, and medical follow-up among individuals testing positive for hepatitis C: National Health and Nutrition Examination Survey 2001-2008. Hepatology 2012;55(6):1652–61.
13. Koretz RL, Brezina M, Polito AJ, et al. Non-A, non-B posttransfusion hepatitis: comparing C and non-C hepatitis. Hepatology 1993;17(3):361–5.
14. Marranconi F, Mecenero V, Pellizzer GP, et al. HCV infection after accidental needlestick injury in health-care workers. Infection 1992;20(2):111.
15. Seeff LB. Hepatitis C from a needlestick injury. Ann Intern Med 1991;115(5):411.
16. Hagan H, Des Jarlais DC, Stern R, et al. HCV synthesis project: preliminary analyses of HCV prevalence in relation to age and duration of injection. Int J Drug Policy 2007;18(5):341–51.
17. Hagan H, Thiede H, Weiss NS, et al. Sharing of drug preparation equipment as a risk factor for hepatitis C. Am J Public Health 2001;91(1):42–6.
18. Lucidarme D, Bruandet A, Ilef D, et al. Incidence and risk factors of HCV and HIV infections in a cohort of intravenous drug users in the North and East of France. Epidemiol Infect 2004;132(4):699–708.
19. Garfein RS, Vlahov D, Galai N, et al. Viral infections in short-term injection drug users: the prevalence of the hepatitis C, hepatitis B, human immunodeficiency, and human T-lymphotropic viruses. Am J Public Health 1996;86(5):655–61.
20. CDC. Prevention and control of infections with hepatitis viruses in correctional settings. MMWR Recomm Rep 2003;52(RR-01):1–33.
21. Thompson ND, Perz JF, Moorman AC, et al. Nonhospital health care-associated hepatitis B and C virus transmission: United States, 1998–2008. Ann Intern Med 2009;150(1):33–9.
22. Alter MJ. Occupational exposure to hepatitis C virus: a dilemma. Infect Control Hosp Epidemiol 1994;15(12):742–4.
23. Lanphear BP, Linnemann CC Jr, Cannon CG, et al. Hepatitis C virus infection in healthcare workers: risk of exposure and infection. Infect Control Hosp Epidemiol 1994;15(12):745–50.
24. Puro V, Petrosillo N, Ippolito G. Risk of hepatitis C seroconversion after occupational exposures in health care workers. Italian study group on occupational risk of HIV and other bloodborne infections. Am J Infect Control 1995;23(5):273–7.

25. Mitsui T, Iwano K, Masuko K, et al. Hepatitis C virus infection in medical personnel after needlestick accident. Hepatology 1992;16(5):1109–14.
26. Scheinmann R, Hagan H, Lelutiu-Weinberger C, et al. Non-injection drug use and hepatitis C virus: a systematic review. Drug Alcohol Depend 2007;89(1):1–12.
27. Kamili S, Krawczynski K, McCaustland K, et al. Infectivity of hepatitis C virus in plasma after drying and storing at room temperature. Infect Control Hosp Epidemiol 2007;28(5):519–24.
28. Mast EE, Hwang LY, Seto DS, et al. Risk factors for perinatal transmission of hepatitis C virus (HCV) and the natural history of HCV infection acquired in infancy. J Infect Dis 2005;192(11):1880–9.
29. Thomas DL, Villano SA, Riester KA, et al. Perinatal transmission of hepatitis C virus from human immunodeficiency virus type 1-infected mothers. Women and infants transmission study. J Infect Dis 1998;177(6):1480–8.
30. Alter MJ, Gerety RJ, Smallwood LA, et al. Sporadic non-A, non-B hepatitis: frequency and epidemiology in an urban U.S. population. J Infect Dis 1982; 145(6):886–93.
31. Williams IT, Bell BP, Kuhnert W, et al. Incidence and transmission patterns of acute hepatitis C in the United States, 1982–2006. Arch Intern Med 2011;171(3):242–8.
32. Vandelli C, Renzo F, Romano L, et al. Lack of evidence of sexual transmission of hepatitis C among monogamous couples: results of a 10-year prospective follow-up study. Am J Gastroenterol 2004;99(5):855–9.
33. Balogun MA, Ramsay ME, Parry JV, et al. A national survey of genitourinary medicine clinic attenders provides little evidence of sexual transmission of hepatitis C virus infection. Sex Transm Infect 2003;79(4):301–6.
34. Marincovich B, Castilla J, del Romero J, et al. Absence of hepatitis C virus transmission in a prospective cohort of heterosexual serodiscordant couples. Sex Transm Infect 2003;79(2):160–2.
35. Terrault NA. Sexual activity as a risk factor for hepatitis C. Hepatology 2002; 36(5 Suppl 1):S99–105.
36. Bottieau E, Apers L, Van Esbroeck M, et al. Hepatitis C virus infection in HIV-infected men who have sex with men: sustained rising incidence in Antwerp, Belgium, 2001-2009. Euro Surveill 2010;15(39):19673.
37. van de Laar TJ, van der Bij AK, Prins M, et al. Increase in HCV incidence among men who have sex with men in Amsterdam most likely caused by sexual transmission. J Infect Dis 2007;196(2):230–8.
38. Fox J, Nastouli E, Thomson E, et al. Increasing incidence of acute hepatitis C in individuals diagnosed with primary HIV in the United Kingdom. AIDS 2008;22(5): 666–8.
39. CDC. Sexual transmission of hepatitis C virus among HIV-infected men who have sex with men– New York City, 2005—2010. MMWR Recomm Rep 2011;60(28):945–50.
40. Armstrong GL, Alter MJ, McQuillan GM, et al. The past incidence of hepatitis C virus infection: implications for the future burden of chronic liver disease in the United States. Hepatology 2000;31:777–82.
41. Alter MJ. Epidemiology of hepatitis C. Hepatology 1997;26(Suppl):62S–5S.
42. CDC. Viral hepatitis surveillance, United States, 2009–2011. Available at: http://www.cdc.gov/hepatitis/Statistics/2010Surveillance/index.htm. Accessed June 18, 2012.
43. CDC. Hepatitis C virus infection among adolescents and young adults –Massachusetts, 2002—2009. MMWR Recomm Rep 2011;60(17):537–54.
44. CDC. Notes from the field: hepatitis C virus infections among young adults–rural Wisconsin, 2010. MMWR Recomm Rep 2012;61(19):358.

45. Chak E, Talal A, Sherman K, et al. Hepatitis C virus infection in USA: an estimate of true prevalence. Liver Int 2011;31:1090–101.
46. Kim WR, Terrault NA, Pedersen RA, et al. Trends in waiting list registration for liver transplantation for viral hepatitis in the United States. Gastroenterology 2009; 137(5):1680–6.
47. El-Serag HB. Epidemiology of viral hepatitis and hepatocellular carcinoma. Gastroenterology 2012;142(6):1264–73.
48. Simard EP, Ward EM, Siegel R, et al. Cancers with increasing incidence trends in the United States: 1999 through 2008. CA Cancer J Clin 2012;62:118–28.
49. Freeman AJ, Dore GJ, Law MG, et al. Estimating progression to cirrhosis in chronic hepatitis C virus infection. Hepatology 2001;34(4 Pt 1):809–16.
50. Hassan MM, Frome A, Patt YZ, et al. Rising prevalence of hepatitis C virus infection among patients recently diagnosed with hepatocellular carcinoma in the United States. J Clin Gastroenterol 2002;35(3):266–9.
51. Rein DB, Wittenborn JS, Weinbaum CM, et al. Forecasting the morbidity and mortality associated with prevalent cases of pre-cirrhotic chronic hepatitis C in the United States. Dig Liver Dis 2011;43(1):66–72.
52. Smith BD, Patel N, Beckett GA, et al. Hepatitis C virus antibody prevalence, correlates and predictors among persons born from 1945 through 1965, United States, 1999–2008 [abstract]. San Francisco (CA): American Association for the Study of Liver Disease; 2011.
53. Kanwal F, Hoang T, Kramer JR, et al. Increasing prevalence of HCC and cirrhosis in patients with chronic hepatitis C virus infection. Gastroenterology 2011;140(4): 1182–8.
54. Su J, Brook RA, Kleinman NL, et al. The impact of hepatitis C virus infection on work absence, productivity, and healthcare benefit costs. Hepatology 2010; 52(2):436–42.
55. Davis KL, Mitra D, Medjedovic J, et al. Direct economic burden of chronic hepatitis C virus in a United States managed care population. J Clin Gastroenterol 2011;45(2):17–24.
56. Wong JB, Davis GL, McHutchison JG, et al. Economic and clinical effects of evaluating rapid viral response to peginterferon alfa-2b plus ribavirin for the initial treatment of chronic hepatitis C. Am J Gastroenterol 2003;98(11):2354–62.
57. Sullivan SD, Jensen DM, Bernstein DE, et al. Cost-effectiveness of combination peginterferon alpha-2a and ribavirin compared with interferon alpha-2b and ribavirin in patients with chronic hepatitis C. Am J Gastroenterol 2004;99(8): 1490–6.
58. Lok AS, Gardiner DF, Lawitz E. Preliminary study of two antiviral agents for hepatitis C genotype 1. N Engl J Med 2012;366(3):216–24.
59. Ghany M, Nelson D, Strader D, et al. An update on treatment of genotype 1 chronic hepatitis C virus infection: 2011 practice guideline by the American Association for the Study of Liver Diseases. Hepatology 2011;54(4):1433–44.
60. IOM (Institute of Medicine). Hepatitis and liver cancer: a national strategy for prevention and control of hepatitis B and C. Washington, DC: The National Academies Press; 2010.
61. CDC. Recommendations for prevention and control of hepatitis C virus (HCV) infection and HCV-related chronic disease. MMWR Recomm Rep 1998;47(RR–19): 1–39.
62. CDC. Recommendations for the identification of chronic hepatitis C virus (HCV) among persons born during 1945-1965. MMWR Recomm Rep 2012;61(RR-4): 1–32.

63. Rein DB, Smith BD, Wittenborn JS, et al. The cost-effectiveness of birth-cohort screening for hepatitis C antibody in U.S. primary care settings. Ann Intern Med 2012;156(4):263–70.
64. US Department of Health and Human Services. Combating the silent epidemic of viral hepatitis: action plan for the prevention, care, and treatment of viral hepatitis. Washington, DC: HHS; 2011. p. 1–76.
65. Arora S, Thornton K, Murata G, et al. Outcomes of treatment for hepatitis C virus infection by primary care providers. N Engl J Med 2011;364(23):2199–207.
66. Smith BD, Drobeniuc J, Jewett A, et al. Evaluation of three rapid screening assays for detection of antibodies to hepatitis C virus. J Infect Dis 2011;204(6):825–31.

Hepatitis C Viral Kinetics
The Past, Present, and Future

Anushree Chatterjee, PhD[a,b], Patrick F. Smith, PhD[c],
Alan S. Perelson, PhD[a,*]

KEYWORDS

- Mathematical modeling • Viral kinetics • Direct-acting antiviral agents
- Protease inhibitors • Hepatitis C virus

KEY POINTS

- The future goal for hepatitis C virus (HCV) therapy is an interferon-free treatment, reduced treatment duration, and higher treatment effectiveness for all genotypes, for both treatment-naïve and treatment-experienced patients.
- To achieve these goals, viral kinetic models that incorporate new drug classes, resistance, and combination therapy should be developed.
- This may allow us to further improve the therapeutics of HCV by applying these models in a way that both enhances the development of new drugs and further optimizes the use of approved therapies.
- In the past, mathematical modeling of HCV kinetics has allowed for estimation of crucial parameters associated with treatment and provided relevant biological explanations for HCV kinetics during primary infection as well as during antiviral therapy.
- These models have also been applied in an attempt to improve the success rate and efficiency of drug development, and to optimize the use of currently approved therapies.
- In the future, mathematical modeling will certainly continue to serve as an important tool to quantitatively assess and develop an improved understanding of HCV therapy.

INTRODUCTION

Hepatitis C virus (HCV) is a positive-strand RNA virus of the Flaviviridae family that primarily infects hepatocytes and can lead to liver cirrhosis, hepatocellular carcinoma, liver failure, and liver failure–related death.[1,2] Chronic HCV infection affects nearly 170 million people worldwide.[3] At present, a vaccine for HCV does not exist. Until recently, the standard of care used to treat HCV included a combination of pegylated interferon-α (PEG-IFN) and ribavirin (RBV).[4] Both of these drugs are general inhibitors of viral infection but only 50% or fewer of patients infected with HCV genotype 1 and

[a] Theoretical Biology and Biophysics, Los Alamos National Laboratory, NM 87545, USA;
[b] Center for Nonlinear Studies, Los Alamos National Laboratory, NM 87545, USA; [c] Clinical Pharmacology, Pharma Research and Early Development, Roche, Nutley, NJ, USA
* Corresponding author.
E-mail address: asp@lanl.gov

Clin Liver Dis 17 (2013) 13–26
http://dx.doi.org/10.1016/j.cld.2012.09.003
1089-3261/13/$ – see front matter © 2013 Elsevier Inc. All rights reserved.

treated with PEG-IFN plus RBV achieve a sustained virologic response (SVR), which is defined as the absence of detectable virus at the end of therapy and 6 months later.[5] Research in understanding the mechanisms of HCV replication has led to the development of direct-acting antiviral agents (DAAs) that target specific aspects of the HCV lifecycle.[6]

The, NS3-4A protease, the NS5B RNA-dependent RNA polymerase (RdRp), and the NS5A protein have been extensively studied as drug targets.[7–10] Some examples of NS3-4A protease inhibitors include telaprevir, boceprevir, TMC435, MK-7009, and RG7227 (reviewed in Ciesek and colleagues[7]). Monotherapy with telaprevir, a specific peptidomimetic inhibitor of NS3-4A, has been found to be very effective in suppressing viral loads (nearly 3–4 logs); however, some patients, especially those infected with genotype 1a, exhibit rapid viral breakthrough and the emergence of resistant virus.[11–13] Similarly, boceprevir monotherapy has showed potent antiviral activity.[14] DAAs targeting NS5B include the nucleoside/nucleotide inhibitors (such as NM283, R1626, R7128 and IDX184, reviewed in Thompson and colleagues[10] and Rong and Perelson[15]) and non-nucleoside inhibitors (such as R803, HCV371 and HCV086, reviewed in Thompson and colleagues[10] and Rong and Perelson[15]), which act respectively by direct targeting the catalytic site and via indirect allosteric mechanisms.

DAA-based monotherapy can result in viral breakthrough because of development of drug resistance.[16–18] One mechanism to overcome resistance is to combine DAAs with PEG-IFN+RBV. In the case of the protease inhibitors boceprevir and telaprevir, this approach has been highly effective, yielding SVR rates of approximately 70%, and these combinations have been approved for patient use.[8,19]

Understanding the key mechanisms of action of DAA-based therapy is essential for the development of more-potent drugs and in designing effective IFN-free regimens. Previously, mathematical modeling of HCV infection under therapy has been successful in deciphering the modes of action of IFN, PEG-IFN, and PEG-IFN+RBV by studying the viral dynamics of HCV RNA decline under therapy.[20–23] Mathematical models fit to patient data provided key parameter estimates, such as the HCV half-life, the virus clearance rate, and infected cell life spans, which have been crucial in understanding the disease. Only a few mathematical models have been used to fit DAA treatment data. In this review, we outline the current mathematical models for HCV dynamics under IFN-based and DAA therapy, and future directions.

MODELING IFN ANTIVIRAL THERAPY

A mathematical model, developed by Neumann and colleagues,[20] explained the biphasic HCV RNA decline observed during high-dose daily IFN treatment (**Fig. 1**A). According to the model, IFN blocked viral production from infected cells with an effectiveness, ε, leading to a rapid reduction in viral load as existing virus was cleared from the circulation and not effectively replaced because of the block in virion production. This rapid first phase was then followed by a slower second phase that reflected the loss of infected cells, which because of lower loads were not effectively replaced by de novo infections. Because the parameters in this model have gained widespread use, it is worthwhile to present them in the context of a schematic version of the model (see **Fig. 1**B).

In the model, target cells, T, are infected by virus, V, a process characterized by the rate constant β. Infected cells, I, are lost via a first-order process at rate δ per infected cell. This loss represents cell death as well as possible "cure" through loss of replicative intermediates. Infected cells produce new virus at rate p per cell, and free virions are assumed to be cleared at rate c per virion. Target cells are assumed to be

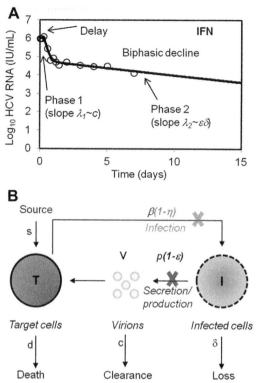

Fig. 1. Viral decline during treatment with IFN. (*A*) A biphasic HCV RNA decline during IFN-α treatment of chronic HCV. (*B*) Schematic representation of the standard viral dynamic model. Treatment may block vRNA production with effectiveness ε, and viral infection by a factor η. *T* and *I* represent target and infected cells, respectively, and *V* represents virus in serum. Target cells are created and die with constant rates *s* and *d*, respectively, and are infected by virus, *V*, with rate constant β. Infected cells, *I*, are lost with rate constant δ and virus, *V*, is cleared from serum with rate constant *c*.

generated at a rate *s* and die at a rate *d* per cell. Later models allow target cells to proliferate.[24] Drug, in this case, IFN, was assumed to act in 2 possible ways: to block new infections with an effectiveness η and/or to block virion production with an effectiveness ε. These effectiveness parameters were assumed to take on values between 0 and 1, with 0 meaning having no effect and 1 meaning 100% effective.

For IFN treatment, fitting patient data under the assumption that the target cell level remained constant for the 14 days of therapy studied, showed that IFN is mainly responsible for blocking virion production, whereas the effect on reducing infection was found to be less significant and difficult to estimate.[20] Because the effect of η on viral load was insignificant compared with the effect of blocking production, η is set to zero in many models. In the Neumann and colleagues[20] model, it was assumed that the dose of drug was high enough that the drug effectiveness could be assumed to be constant over the course of treatment. Thus, this model is sometimes called the constant effectiveness (CE) model.[25]

The CE model, when fitted to HCV RNA data after initiation of IFN treatment, provided an estimate of the mean virion clearance rate *c* of approximately 6 d^{-1},[20] corresponding to a mean viral half-life in serum of about 2.7 hours. Estimates for ε and δ have been found to be dependent on the HCV genotype, ethnicity, polymorphism in the interleukin 28 B (IL28B), baseline viral load, baseline inducible protein 10 (IP-10) levels, and histologic factors,[26–30] but for patients with genotype 1, high daily doses of 10 or 15 million international units (MIU) of standard IFN lead to effectiveness estimates of ε of approximately 0.95.[20]

The mathematical form of the "standard" model shown in **Fig. 1B** is valid when the constant drug effectiveness assumption holds, such as in the case of high-dose daily administration of IFN. However, in cases such as PEG-IFN therapy, in which the drug is administered once a week, the concentration of drug initially increases and then decreases over the dosing interval, resulting in fluctuations in HCV RNA levels.[25,31,32] Under these circumstances, the CE assumption fails, and such conditions are better described by a varying effectiveness (VE) model based on the pharmacokinetic/pharmacodynamic (PK/PD) characteristics of the drugs used.[25] In the VE model, the drug effectiveness is considered to vary over time. These models have been reviewed in Shudo and colleagues[25] and Guedj and colleagues.[33]

THE PRESENT: MODELING HCV RNA DECLINE DURING DAA-BASED THERAPY
Modeling HCV RNA Decline During Telaprevir-Based Therapy

During treatment with telaprevir (TVR), an HCV NS3-4A protease inhibitor, a biphasic viral decline is also observed (**Fig. 2A**). Mathematical models when fit to data from 44 patients treated with TVR, showed a more rapid second-phase decline than seen previously with IFN-based therapies.[34] To quantify the HCV dynamics, Adiwajaya and colleagues[34] used a version of the standard (CE) model to fit the early phase of treatment (first 3 days), a period presumed short enough to justify neglecting the influence of resistant variants (see **Fig. 1B**). The model estimated the median infected cell clearance rate to be $\delta = 1.2 \ \mathrm{d}^{-1}$, which was roughly 10 times higher than that reported for IFN-based treatment. Additionally, the median δ for TVR monotherapy was more than twice that of TVR+PEG-IFN-α2a+RBV treatment. This is also 3 to 4 times higher than that reported for another protease inhibitor BILN-2061. On the other hand, estimates for the plasma virion clearance rate, c, were found to be similar to that reported for PEG-IFN-α2a+RBV and BILN-2061–based regimens, and about twofold higher compared with IFN-α2b–based and PEG-IFN-α2a–based regimen.[35]

Guedj and Perelson[36] fit the same patient data using a VE model, instead of the CE model to account for time taken for TVR concentration in plasma to reach maximum levels. Treatment effectiveness ε was allowed to vary over time, as shown in **Fig. 2B**, where ε_1 and ε_2 are the initial and final treatment effectiveness ($\varepsilon_2 > \varepsilon_1$), respectively, and k is rate of change of effectiveness. Interestingly, no significant difference was found for drug effectiveness parameters (k, ε_1 and ε_2) and viral dynamics when comparing TVR+PEG-IFN-α2a with TVR monotherapy. The model estimated the initial treatment effectiveness of $\varepsilon_1 = 0.974$, defined as the effectiveness at the first time a viral load decline could be discerned, and a significantly higher final treatment effectiveness of $\varepsilon_2 = 0.999$. The mean infected cell loss rate was estimated to be $\delta = 0.58 \ \mathrm{d}^{-1}$ for patients receiving monotherapy and $\delta = 0.57 \ \mathrm{d}^{-1}$ for patients receiving combination therapy (TVR+PEG-IFN), which was significantly lower than that estimated by the CE model ($\delta = 1.2 \ \mathrm{d}^{-1}$).[34] Both CE[34] and VE[36] models indicated that TVR exhibits a rapid second-phase decrease when compared with IFN-based treatments.

Typically, the second-phase decline is attributed to infected cell death δ. Interestingly, a linear correlation between δ and the log-transformed treatment effectiveness $(1-\varepsilon_2)$ was found (see **Fig. 2C**), indicating that high effectiveness not only generated

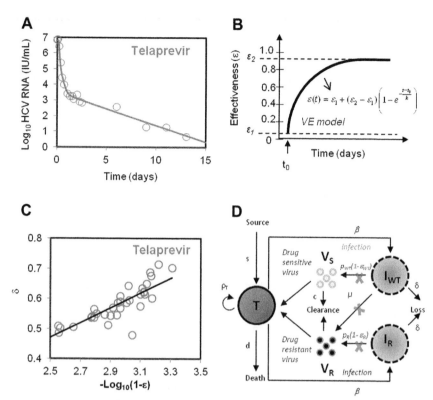

Fig. 2. Mathematical modeling of HCV kinetics during treatment with protease inhibitor telaprevir. (A) A biphasic viral decline of measured HCV RNA during treatment with telaprevir+IFN is observed. (B) The effectiveness of drug varying over time using VE models. (C) The rate of loss of infected liver cells is linearly correlated with log-transformed drug effectiveness, ε_2. (D) Schematic representation of 2-strain viral dynamic model for drug-sensitive (V_S) and drug-resistant virus (V_R); ρ_T is the proliferation rate of target cells, p_S and p_R are the production rate of drug-sensitive and drug-resistant virus strains respectively. Drug effectiveness in reducing viral production from drug-sensitive and drug-resistant strains is denoted by ε_S and ε_R respectively, and μ is the rate of mutation from drug-sensitive to drug-resistant strain. ([D] Adapted from Rong L, Dahari H, Ribeiro RM, et al. Rapid emergence of protease inhibitor resistance in hepatitis C virus. Sci Transl Med 2010;2(30):30ra32; with permission.)

a more profound first-phase decline but also a faster second-phase decline. As a result, the time required for achieving less than 1 virion in the extracellular volume or less than 1 infected cell in the liver, was predicted to be considerably shortened with TVR as compared with IFN-based treatments. The VE model predicted that in fully compliant patients with no evidence of drug resistance, the threshold of less than 1 virion could be achieved within 7 and 8 weeks for 95% and 99% of patients respectively. Although this time frame is significantly shorter than currently recommended, the emergence of drug resistance could further extend the needed treatment duration.

Viral Breakthrough During Telaprevir Monotherapy

Viral breakthrough hinders the applicability of current protease inhibitors as monotherapy agents.[11,17,37,38] This is primarily because of the high replication rate of HCV and the high error rate of HCV RdRp (estimated as 2.5×10^{-5} per base per generation[39]). Because DAAs target specific structural properties of HCV proteins, often a single point mutation is sufficient to confer resistance.[15] For example, the single mutations T54A, V36A/M, R155K/T, and A156V/T confer different degrees of TVR resistance.[40] Some studies have monitored the selection and kinetics of drug-resistant HCV variants.[11–13,17,40–42] A 14-day monotherapy treatment with TVR showed that all 4 treated patients with genotype 1a developed resistance,[13] with approximately 5% to 20% of the viral pool consisting of drug-resistant variants as early as day 2 of treatment.

Because of the importance of understanding drug resistance to DAAs, mathematical models have been used to quantify the emergence and buildup of drug-resistant variants.[29,37,43] Rong and colleagues[37] used a model (see **Fig. 2**D) that considered 2 viral strains, drug sensitive and drug resistant, to track the development of drug resistance during TVR treatment. The model assumed low levels of drug-resistant variants existed before the start of the treatment, with their levels determined by "mutation-selection balance" (ie, the HCV RdRp error rate and the fitness of the variant).[44] The high frequency of drug-resistant variants detected in the patients with genotype 1a on day 2 of therapy could be explained by the profound first-phase decline in the drug-sensitive population, in essence revealing the preexisting drug-resistant variants. The rapid growth of the resistant variants observed after day 2 required "replication space." In the model, this replication space was provided by the proliferation of target cells. There are other possible sources of replication space, such as growth in cells already infected by drug-sensitive virus or the loss of an IFN-induced antiviral state in cells previously protected by the endogenous IFN response. We expect that as viral loads decline because of DAA therapy, endogenous IFN responses will decline as well. Whether this occurs sufficiently rapidly to explain the observed growth of the resistant variants remains to be resolved.

The Rong and colleagues'[37] model that included only 2 viral strains was purposely kept simple. More complex models that kept track of multiple resistant variants, each with different fitness and different drug sensitivity, were developed by Adiwijaya and colleagues[43] and Rong and colleagues.[45] The Adiwijaya and colleagues' model[43] was fit to data from telaprevir clinical trials and explained the dynamics of the various resistant variants observed in the patient data. The Rong and colleagues' model[45] studied from a more mathematical perspective the properties of multistrain systems and explored the role of mutation versus preexistence of resistant strains and the specific viral properties that determine variant frequency. Both models showed that the mere presence of resistant variants does not mean that they will grow and cause viral rebound. The fitness and drug sensitivity of the variants, as well as the properties of the species they are competing with within the patient, may all be needed to predict patient outcome. A more practical approach to the drug-resistance problem is to use combination therapy that provides a high barrier to resistance. Thus, modeling has also focused on determining the viral kinetic properties and modes of action of other classes of antiviral agents.

Modeling HCV Kinetics with Mericitabine (RG7128)

Mericitabine is an oral cytidine nucleoside that exhibits a strong antiviral effectiveness against HCV RNA polymerase across all genotypes.[46] On cellular uptake, mericitabine is converted to cytidine monophosphate, which is further phosphorylated intracellularly to the active cytidine triphosphate and uridine triphosphate forms. Motivated by the need of the active triphosphates to accumulate intracellularly, the variable effectiveness model was used by Guedj and colleagues[47] to fit data from 32 IFN-treatment experienced patients infected by HCV-genotype 1 (**Fig. 3**A). In this study,

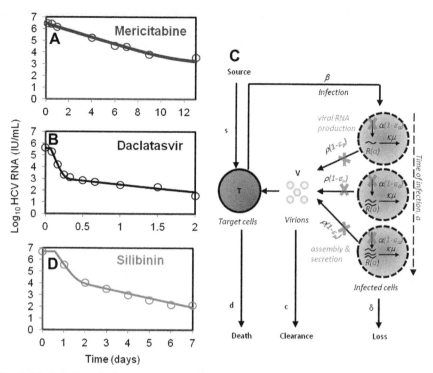

Fig. 3. Viral decline during treatment with various DAAs and an improved mathematical model of HCV kinetics. (*A, B*) A monophasic decline of measured HCV RNA with mericitabine monotherapy (*A*), and a biphasic decline with daclatasvir (*B*) is observed. (*C*) Schematic representation of the modified model for fitting early HCV viral load decline during treatment with daclatasvir. Here, intracellular HCV RNA (vRNA) is denoted by R; production, degradation, and assembly/secretion occur at rates α, μ, and ρ, respectively. Treatment may block vRNA production with effectiveness ε_α, and/or virion assembly/secretion with effectiveness ε_s and/or enhance the degradation rate (μ) of vRNA by a factor κ. (*D*) A biphasic viral decline of measured HCV RNA during treatment with silibinin monotherapy is observed.

mericitabine was given for 14 days to 4 groups of patients at dosages of 750 mg once daily (750 mg every day), 1500 mg once daily (1500 mg every day), 750 mg twice daily (750 mg twice a day), and 1500 mg twice daily (1500 mg twice a day).

The effectiveness of mericitabine was found to increase during treatment in a dose-dependent manner, with mean final effectiveness $\varepsilon_2 = 0.86$ (for 750 mg every day) and $\varepsilon_2 = 0.94$ (for 1500 mg every day), and a significantly higher mean effectiveness for the twice-a-day groups, $\varepsilon_2 = 0.98$ (for 750 mg twice a day) and $\varepsilon_2 = 0.998$ (for 1500 mg twice a day). Not surprisingly, the rate at which the treatment effectiveness built up (parameter k in equation shown in **Fig. 2B**) was found to be significantly higher for patients in the twice-a-day dosing groups than in the patients given drug once a day. With twice-a-day dosing it took 2.9 days on average for 90% of the final effectiveness to be attained and 6.5 days to reach 99% of the final effectiveness.[47] Because of the slow buildup of effectiveness, all patients treated with mericitabine showed a slow viral decline within the first 4 days of treatment when compared with patients treated with IFN, a protease inhibitor, or an NS5A inhibitor.[34,36] In patients who needed additional time to reach high levels of antiviral effectiveness, there was a slower initial rate of viral decline, with 12 patients exhibiting a single phase of monotonic decline, rather than the typical biphasic decline usually observed with IFN or protease inhibitor therapy. The mean value of δ was 0.023 d^{-1}, with no significant differences among the various treatment groups. This value is much lower than that reported for IFN-based therapy and may be biased, as all these patients failed prior IFN-based therapy and hence may have slow second-phase declines. Interestingly, unlike other DAAs, viral breakthrough was not reported at the end of treatment. This suggests that, even though mericitabine may act slowly via a monophasic manner, it could be combined with other DAAs to develop effective treatments.

Viral Kinetics During Treatment with the NS5A Inhibitor Daclatsvir (BMS-79002)

The first-in-class inhibitor of the nonstructural NS5A protein of HCV, daclatasvir, is very effective and can decrease HCV RNA levels by as much as 3 orders of magnitude within 12 hours postdosing (see **Fig. 3B**)[48]; however, the mechanism(s) of action of daclatasvir remain unclear. To understand the action of daclatasvir, Guedj and colleagues (submitted for publication) developed a multilevel model, which accounted for the dynamics of intracellular genomic viral RNA (vRNA) so as to incorporate the steps of intracellular viral replication directly targeted by DAAs (see **Fig. 3C**).

In this model, vRNA was assumed to be produced at a constant rate α, removed at a constant rate μ, and exported into the circulation as virions at rate ρ per vRNA. The model incorporates the age of an infected cell, denoted a, which is defined as the time elapsed postinfection. As time after infection increases, vRNA should accumulate in the infected cell and this new model keeps track of this. The model allows for 3 possible effects of daclatasvir: (1) blocking of vRNA production with effectiveness ε_α, (2) blocking vRNA assembly into virions and/or secretion with effectiveness ε_p, and (3) enhancement of vRNA degradation (denoted as μ) by a factor $\kappa>1$. The model was fit to patient data from 5 subjects receiving a single dose of 10 or 100 mg of daclatasvir. The model was also fit to data from 20 patients on IFN therapy, and revealed that daclatasvir appeared to have significant activity in blocking both viral assembly/secretion and vRNA replication, whereas IFN mainly affected vRNA replication (Guedj and colleagues, submitted for publication). Further, the first-phase decay observed with daclatasvir was very rapid and suggested that HCV may have a half-life as short as 45 minutes. This fast decay can be deduced from the HCV RNA decay shown in **Fig. 1** of Gao and colleagues,[48] without the use of any modeling, and is comparable to the half-life reported for HIV.[49]

Modeling the Viral Kinetics During Treatment with Silibinin

Silibinin, the active component of Legalon SIL, has exhibited significant antiviral activity against HCV genotypes 1 and 4. SVR has been reported in a patient treated with SIL monotherapy for 1 week, followed by 15 weeks of PEG+RBV. Despite its success, the mode of action of SIL is not clearly understood. Ahmed-Belkacem and colleagues,[50] based on in vitro studies, showed that the mode of action of SIL was inhibiting the HCV NS5B-RdRp, whereas Wagoner and colleagues,[51,52] based on in vivo data, suggested silibinin blocks infection and cell-to-cell spread.

Guedj and colleagues[27] modeled HCV RNA kinetics measured (once per day) in 25 patients, treated for 1 week with SIL monotherapy, with dosages of 10, 15, and 20 mg/kg, as reported in Ferenci and colleagues.[53] Using the standard model to fit the data yielded a dose-dependent effectiveness ($\varepsilon = 0.69$ for the 10 + 15 mg/kg group and $\varepsilon = 0.91$ for the 20 mg/kg group). The infected cell loss rate was estimated at $\delta = 0.91$ d^{-1}, which is higher than that reported for IFN-based therapy.[20,34]

Interestingly, the data indicated that 40% of patients showed a monophasic viral RNA decline (see **Fig. 3**D). A higher infected cell loss rate was estimated for monophasic patients ($\delta = 1.1$ d^{-1}) compared with patients with a biphasic decline ($\delta = 0.83$ d^{-1}), although both groups showed a similar viral decline rate between days 2 and 7. A model assuming SIL inhibits viral infection as well as viral production estimated an effectiveness in blocking infection of $\eta = 0.6$ and yielded a statistically improved fit to patient data. This analysis suggested that SIL potentially acts via both these modes in vivo, with blocking viral production being the more pronounced mode of action, consistent with experimental data.[50–52,54]

Impact of Viral Kinetic Modeling on Therapeutics and Drug Development

The insights gained from viral kinetic modeling have contributed both to improving our understanding of the treatment of patients with HCV, as well as to the development of new antivirals. The Neumann and colleagues'[20] model for IFN, described previously, was extended by Dahari and colleagues[24] and further applied to the prediction of treatment outcomes. Snoeck and colleagues[55] applied HCV viral kinetic modeling to a large database of more than 2000 patients with clinical outcomes who were treated with PEG-IFN-α-2a and RBV, using nonlinear mixed effects modeling. Introducing the concept of a "cure boundary," the investigators were able to describe and predict therapeutic outcomes with a high degree of accuracy. This model has further been used to simulate therapeutic outcomes of alternative PEG-IFN-α-2a dosing regimens and in special patient populations, facilitating clinical trial design and support of dose recommendations for drug labeling. This PEG-IFN-α-2a–based model has been further extended to incorporate the protease inhibitor danoprevir, and qualified to simulate clinical trial outcomes of triple combination therapy (PEG-IFN-α-2a plus danoprevir/ritonavir and RBV) regimens including different danoprevir doses and treatment durations (Roche, unpublished data).

Viral kinetic modeling has also been used to facilitate the design of early-phase clinical trials, both as a translational tool to bridge preclinical data to human trials, and to generate hypotheses for optimizing dosing regimens of DAAs, which can then be evaluated in patients. For example, the varying effectiveness of the viral kinetic model for mericitabine, described previously,[47] has led to the hypothesis that a short lead-in dosing strategy of nucleoside polymerase inhibitors, when given in combination with DAAs with a low barrier to resistance, may enhance the ability of the nucleoside to protect against resistance. This strategy is currently being tested in 2 clinical trials involving both mericitabine and GS-7977. The results of the trials will determine whether the benefit of this approach translates into a clinically meaningful difference.

An example of a translational use of HCV viral kinetic modeling is provided by the Toll-like receptor 7 (TLR7) agonist PF-04878691.[56] In this example, an HCV viral kinetic model was used to predict the antiviral activity of a TLR7 agonist, based on the observed level of stimulation of the IFN system with various dosing regimens of PF-0487691 in animals. Translational pharmacokinetic-pharmacodynamic modeling facilitated the selection of the first human doses and the estimation of the likely human effective dose.[56] Once healthy volunteer data were available, the model was updated with human clinical data and used to support a go/no-go decision with regard to further clinical development.[57]

HCV viral kinetic modeling has also been applied to drug discovery and early drug development. Reddy and colleagues[58] described the identification of key parameters associated with the clinical potency of HCV protease inhibitors and non-nucleoside polymerase inhibitors. These model-based relationships were used to optimize the nomination of compounds for consideration to move into clinical development, and to facilitate the design of phase I clinical trials, by improving the prediction of clinically effective doses.

THE FUTURE: MODELING COMBINATION THERAPY OF DAAS AND ROLE OF INTRACELLULAR FACTORS DURING DAA TREATMENT

Currently DAA therapy with telaprevir or boceprevir involves concomitant administration of PEG-IFN and RBV, for both treatment-naïve and treatment-experienced patients. Although significant improvement in the treatment outcomes have been observed, the underlying limitation of tolerability and efficacy issues associated with IFN-based treatment highlight the need to switch to DAA combination therapy in the future. In the first of its kind study, INFORM-1 provided proof-of-concept that combination of 2 different DAAs can result in successful treatment outcome.[59] In this study, 2 different DAAs, danoprevir, a NS3/4A protease inhibitor,[60] and mericitabine, a nucleoside inhibitor, were administered to patients without concomitant use of IFN or RBV. Danoprevir monotherapy has shown potent activity against HCV[60]; however, similar to other protease inhibitors, has shown emergence of viral breakthrough. The INFORM-1 study showed that with combination therapy a significant 5-log reduction in viral load over a period of 14 days could be achieved, in addition to no viral breakthrough being reported. The success of INFORM-1 has led to several phase-2 trials that have combined various DAAs (summarized in Gane[61]).

So far, mathematical models for IFN-free DAA combination therapy have not been reported. Although the conceptual framework of the biphasic model has brought valuable insights into the origin of the typical viral decline during standard high-dose daily IFN and has been fairly successful in explaining DAA+IFN-based treatments, extensions of this model are needed to understand other observed patterns of viral decline and the response to DAAs. Especially because DAAs act via targeting specific mechanisms during HCV replication, the current models need to be refined to include the pertinent biology. There is still lack of information about hepatocyte kinetics as well as understanding of the intracellular viral RNA replication dynamics. Dahari and colleagues[62] developed a mathematical model describing the dynamics of intracellular HCV replication, providing the first step toward developing a detailed model for HCV replication that can serve as an important tool for evaluating new antivirals. An important aspect of combination therapy is to optimize the number and type of DAAs to achieve high rates of SVR as well as reduced treatment duration.

Additional advances are also needed in the development of viral kinetic models that evaluate the role of host factors that have been shown to influence treatment outcome, such as cyclophilin A,[63] IP-10,[64] and IL28B polymorphism.[65] Until now, most of the DAA-based modeling efforts have been focused on protease inhibitors and NS5A and NS5B nucleoside inhibitors. Mathematical models describing viral kinetics during treatment with entry inhibitors, such as cyanovirin-N,[66] and non-nucleoside inhibitors of HCV RdRp, such as setrobuvir,[67] BI 2027127,[68] and GS-6620,[69] or host factor inhibitors, such as alisporivir,[70] have yet to be explored.

SUMMARY

The future goal for HCV therapy is an IFN-free treatment, reduced treatment duration, and higher treatment effectiveness for all genotypes, for both treatment-naïve and treatment-experienced patients. To achieve these goals, viral kinetic models that incorporate new drug classes, resistance, and combination therapy should be developed. This may allow us to further improve the therapeutics of HCV by applying these models in a way that both enhances the development of new drugs and further optimizes the use of approved therapies. In the past, mathematical modeling of HCV kinetics has allowed for estimation of crucial parameters associated with treatment and provided relevant biological explanations for HCV kinetics during primary infection as well as during antiviral therapy. These models have also been applied in an attempt to improve the success rate and efficiency of drug development, and to optimize the use of currently approved therapies. In the future, mathematical modeling will certainly continue to serve as an important tool to quantitatively assess and develop an improved understanding of HCV therapy.

ACKNOWLEDGMENTS

This work was performed under the auspices of the US Department of Energy under contract DE-AC52-06NA25396, and supported by NIH grants AI028433, P20-RR018754, R34-HL109334, AI078881, the National Center for Research Resources and the Office of Research Infrastructure Programs through grant 8R01-OD011095-21 (ASP), and Roche Inc. We also acknowledge the Los Alamos National Laboratory LDRD (Laboratory Directed Research and Development) Program for providing partial funding for A.C.

REFERENCES

1. Hoofnagle JH. Course and outcome of hepatitis C. Hepatology 2002;36(5):S21–9.
2. Lindenbach BD, Rice CM. Unravelling hepatitis C virus replication from genome to function. Nature 2005;436(7053):933–8.
3. Davis GL, Albright JE, Cook SF, et al. Projecting future complications of chronic hepatitis C in the United States. Liver Transpl 2003;9(4):331–8.
4. McHutchison JG, Lawitz EJ, Shiffman ML, et al. Peginterferon alfa-2b or alfa-2a with ribavirin for treatment of hepatitis C infection. N Engl J Med 2009;361(6):580–93.
5. Abdelmalek MF, Firpi RJ, Soldevila-Pico C, et al. Sustained viral response to interferon and ribavirin in liver transplant recipients with recurrent hepatitis C. Liver Transpl 2004;10(2):199–207.
6. TenCate V, Sainz BJ, Cotler SJ, et al. Potential treatment options and future research to increase hepatitis C virus treatment response rate. Hepat Med 2010;2:125–45.
7. Ciesek S, von Hahn T, Manns MP. Second-wave protease inhibitors: choosing an heir. Clin Liver Dis 2011;15(3):597–609.
8. Hézode C, Forestier N, Dusheiko G, et al. Telaprevir and peginterferon with or without ribavirin for chronic HCV infection. N Engl J Med 2009;360(18):1839–50.
9. Pawlotsky JM. Treatment failure and resistance with direct-acting antiviral drugs against hepatitis C virus. Hepatology 2011;53(5):1742–51.
10. Thompson A, Patel K, Tillman H, et al. Directly acting antivirals for the treatment of patients with hepatitis C infection: a clinical development update addressing key future challenges. J Hepatol 2009;50(1):184–94.
11. De Meyer SM, Dierynck I, Ghys A, et al. Similar incidence of virological failure and emergence of resistance with or without a lead-in: results of a telaprevir Phase 3 study in patients who did not achieve SVR with prior Peg-IFN/RBV treatment. Antivir Ther 2011;16(4):A25.
12. Hiraga N, Imamura M, Abe H, et al. Rapid emergence of telaprevir resistant hepatitis C virus strain from wildtype clone in vivo. Hepatology 2011;54(3):781–8.
13. Kieffer TL, Sarrazin C, Miller JS, et al. Telaprevir and pegylated interferon-alpha-2a inhibit wild-type and resistant genotype 1 hepatitis C virus replication in patients. Hepatology 2007;46(3):631–9.

14. Malcolm BA, Liu R, Lahser F, et al. SCH 503034, a mechanism-based inhibitor of hepatitis C virus NS3 protease, suppresses polyprotein maturation and enhances the antiviral activity of alpha interferon in replicon cells. Antimicrob Agents Chemother 2006;50(3):1013–20.

15. Rong L, Perelson AS. Treatment of hepatitis C virus infection with interferon and small molecule direct antivirals: viral kinetics and modeling. Crit Rev Immunol 2010;30(2):131–48.

16. Bartels DJ, Zhou Y, Zhang EZ, et al. Natural prevalence of hepatitis C virus variants with decreased sensitivity to NS3/4A protease inhibitors in treatment-naive subjects. J Infect Dis 2008;198(6):800–7.

17. Lin C, Gates CA, Rao BG, et al. In vitro studies of cross-resistance mutations against two hepatitis C virus serine protease inhibitors, VX-950 and BILN 2061. J Biol Chem 2005;280(44):36784–91.

18. Nettles RE, Gao M, Bifano M, et al. Multiple ascending dose study of BMS-790052, a nonstructural protein 5A replication complex inhibitor, in patients infected with hepatitis C virus genotype 1. Hepatology 2011;54(6):1956–65.

19. Poordad F, McCone J, Bacon BR, et al. Boceprevir for untreated chronic HCV genotype 1 infection. N Engl J Med 2011;364(13):1195–206.

20. Neumann AU, Lam NP, Dahari H, et al. Hepatitis C viral dynamics in vivo and the antiviral efficacy of interferon-alpha therapy. Science 1998;282(5386):103–7.

21. Perelson AS, Neumann AU, Markowitz M, et al. HIV-1 dynamics in vivo: virion clearance rate, infected cell life-span, and viral generation time. Science 1996; 271(5255):1582–6.

22. Dixit NM, Layden-Almer JE, Layden TJ, et al. Modelling how ribavirin improves interferon response rates in hepatitis C virus infection. Nature 2004;432(7019): 922–4.

23. Perelson AS, Essunger P, Cao YZ, et al. Decay characteristics of HIV-1-infected compartments during combination therapy. Nature 1997;387(6629):188–91.

24. Dahari H, Lo A, Ribeiro RM, et al. Modeling hepatitis C virus dynamics: liver regeneration and critical drug efficacy. J Theor Biol 2007;247(2):371–81.

25. Shudo E, Ribeiro RM, Perelson AS. Modeling HCV kinetics under therapy using PK and PD information. Expert Opin Drug Metab Toxicol 2009;5(3):321–32.

26. Dahari H, Guedj J, Perelson A, et al. Hepatitis C viral kinetics in the era of direct acting antiviral agents and interleukin-28B. Curr Hepat Rep 2011;10(3):214–27.

27. Guedj J, Dahari H, Pohl RT, et al. Understanding silibinin's modes of action against HCV using viral kinetic modeling. J Hepatol 2012;56:1019–24.

28. Ribeiro RM, Layden-Almer J, Powers KA, et al. Dynamics of alanine aminotransferase during hepatitis C virus treatment. Hepatology 2003;38(2):509–17.

29. Guedj J, Neumann AU. Understanding hepatitis C viral dynamics with direct-acting antiviral agents due to the interplay between intracellular replication and cellular infection dynamics. J Theor Biol 2010;267(3):330–40.

30. Guedj H, Guedj J, Negro F, et al. The impact of fibrosis and steatosis on early viral kinetics in HCV genotype 1 infected patients treated with PEG-IFN-alfa-2a and ribavirin. J Viral Hepat 2012;19(7):1365–2893.

31. Welling PG. Pharmacokinetics: processes and mathematics. ACS (American Chemical Society) Monograph 1986;185:XIV+290P.

32. Talal AH, Ribeiro RM, Powers KA, et al. Pharmacodynamics of PEG-IFN alpha differentiate HIV/HCV coinfected sustained virological responders from nonresponders. Hepatology 2006;43(5):943–53.

33. Guedj J, Rong L, Dahari H, et al. A perspective on modelling hepatitis C virus infection. J Viral Hepat 2010;17(12):825–33.

34. Adiwijaya BS, Hare B, Caron PR, et al. Rapid decrease of wild-type hepatitis C virus on telaprevir treatment. Antivir Ther 2009;14(4):591–5.
35. Hinrichsen H, Benhamou Y, Wedemeyer H, et al. Short-term antiviral efficacy of BILN 2061, a hepatitis C virus serine protease inhibitor, in hepatitis C genotype 1 patients. Gastroenterology 2004;127(5):1347–55.
36. Guedj J, Perelson AS. Second-phase hepatitis C virus RNA decline during telaprevir-based therapy increases with drug effectiveness: implications for treatment duration. Hepatology 2011;53(6):1801–8.
37. Rong L, Dahari H, Ribeiro RM, et al. Rapid emergence of protease inhibitor resistance in hepatitis C virus. Sci Transl Med 2010;2(30):30ra32.
38. Tong X, Bogen S, Chase R, et al. Characterization of resistance mutations against HCV ketoamide protease inhibitors. Antiviral Res 2008;77(3):177–85.
39. Ribeiro RM, Li H, Wang S, et al. Quantifying the diversification of hepatitis C virus (HCV) during primary infection: estimates of the in vivo mutation rate. PLoS Pathog 2012;8(8):e1002881.
40. Sarrazin C, Kieffer TL, Bartels D, et al. Dynamic hepatitis C virus genotypic and phenotypic changes in patients treated with the protease inhibitor telaprevir. Gastroenterology 2007;132(5):1767–77.
41. Kieffer TL, De Meyer S, Bartels DJ, et al. Clinical virology findings from treatment-naive and treatment-experienced genotype 1 HCV patients receiving telaprevir/peginterferon/ribavirin in Phase 3 clinical trials. Antivir Ther 2011;16(4):A27.
42. Kieffer T, Zhou Y, Zhang E, et al. Evaluation of viral variants during a Phase 2 study (PROVE2) of telaprevir with peginterferon alfa-2a and ribavirin in treatment-naive HCV genotype I-infected patients. Hepatology 2007;46(4):862A.
43. Adiwijaya BS, Herrmann E, Hare B, et al. A multi-variant, viral dynamic model of genotype 1 HCV to assess the in vivo evolution of protease-inhibitor resistant variants. PLoS Comput Biol 2010;6(4):e1000745.
44. Domingo E. Biological significance of viral quasispecies. Viral Hepatitis Rev 1996;2:247–61.
45. Rong L, Ribeiro RM, Perelson AS. Modeling quasispecies and drug resistance in hepatitis C patients treated with a protease inhibitor. Bull Math Biol 2012;74: 1789–817.
46. Reddy R, Rodriguez-Torres M, Gane E, et al. Antiviral activity, pharmacokinetics, safety and tolerability of R7128, a novel nucleoside HCV RNA polymerase inhibitor, following multiple, ascending, oral doses in patients with HCV genotype 1 infection who have failed prior interferon therapy. Hepatology 2007;46(4):862A–3A.
47. Guedj J, Dahari H, Shudo E, et al. Hepatitis C viral kinetics with the nucleoside polymerase inhibitor mericitabine (RG7128). Hepatology 2012;55:1030–7.
48. Gao M, Nettles RE, Belema M, et al. Chemical genetics strategy identifies an HCV NS5A inhibitor with a potent clinical effect. Nature 2010;465(7294):96–108.
49. Ramratnam B, Bonhoeffer S, Binley J, et al. Rapid production and clearance of HIV-1 and hepatitis C virus assessed by large volume plasma apheresis. Lancet 1999;354(9192):1782–5.
50. Ahmed-Belkacem A, Ahnou N, Barbotte L, et al. Silibinin and related compounds are direct inhibitors of hepatitis C virus RNA-dependent RNA polymerase. Gastroenterology 2010;138(3):1112–22.
51. Wagoner J, Morishima C, Graf TN, et al. Differential in vitro effects of intravenous versus oral formulations of silibinin on the HCV life cycle and inflammation. PLoS One 2011;6(1):e16464.
52. Wagoner J, Negash A, Kane OJ, et al. Multiple effects of silymarin on the hepatitis C virus lifecycle. Hepatology 2010;51(6):1912–21.

53. Ferenci P, Scherzer TM, Kerschner H, et al. Silibinin is a potent antiviral agent in patients with chronic hepatitis C not responding to pegylated interferon/ribavirin therapy. Gastroenterology 2008;135(5):1561–7.
54. Polyak SJ, Morishima C, Shuhart MC, et al. Inhibition of T-cell inflammatory cytokines, hepatocyte NF-kappa B signaling, and HCV infection by standardized silymarin. Gastroenterology 2007;132(5):1925–36.
55. Snoeck E, Chanu P, Lavielle M, et al. A comprehensive hepatitis C viral kinetic model explaining cure. Clin Pharmacol Ther 2010;87(6):706–13.
56. Benson N, de Jongh J, Duckworth JD, et al. Pharmacokinetic-pharmacodynamic modeling of alpha interferon response induced by a Toll-like 7 receptor agonist in mice. Antimicrob Agents Chemother 2010;54(3):1179–85.
57. Jones HM, Chan PL, van der Graaf PH, et al. Use of modelling and simulation techniques to support decision making on the progression of PF-04878691, a TLR7 agonist being developed for hepatitis C. Br J Clin Pharmacol 2012;73(1):77–92.
58. Reddy MB, Morcos PN, Le Pogam S, et al. Pharmacokinetic/pharmacodynamic predictors of clinical potency for hepatitis C virus nonnucleoside polymerase and protease inhibitors. Antimicrob Agents Chemother 2012;56(6):3144–56.
59. Gane EJ, Roberts SK, Stedman CA, et al. Oral combination therapy with a nucleoside polymerase inhibitor (RG7128) and danoprevir for chronic hepatitis C genotype 1 infection (INFORM-1): a randomised, double-blind, placebo-controlled, dose-escalation trial. Lancet 2010;376(9751):1467–75.
60. Forestier N, Larrey D, Guyader D, et al. Treatment of chronic hepatitis C patients with the NS3/4A protease inhibitor danoprevir (ITMN-191/RG7227) leads to robust reductions in viral RNA: a phase 1b multiple ascending dose study. J Hepatol 2011;54(6):1130–6.
61. Gane E. Future hepatitis C virus treatment: interferon-sparing combinations. Liver Int 2011;31:62–7.
62. Dahari H, Ribeiro RM, Rice CM, et al. Mathematical modeling of subgenomic hepatitis C virus replication in Huh-7 cells. J Virol 2007;81(2):750–60.
63. Yang F, Robotham JM, Nelson HB, et al. Cyclophilin A is an essential cofactor for hepatitis C virus infection and the principal mediator of cyclosporine resistance in vitro. J Virol 2008;82(11):5269–78.
64. Lagging M, Romero AI, Westin J, et al. IP-10 predicts viral response and therapeutic outcome in difficult-to-treat patients with HCV genotype 1 infection. Hepatology 2006;44(6):1617–25.
65. Thomas DL, Thio CL, Martin MP, et al. Genetic variation in IL28B and spontaneous clearance of hepatitis C virus. Nature 2009;461(7265):798–801.
66. Helle F, Wychowski C, Vu-Dac N, et al. Cyanovirin-N Inhibits hepatitis C virus entry by binding to envelope protein glycans. J Biol Chem 2006;281(35):25177–83.
67. Lawitz E, Rodriguez-Torres M, DeMico M, et al. Antiviral activity of ANA598, a potent non-nucleoside polymerase inhibitor, in chronic hepatitis C patients. J Hepatol 2009;50:S384.
68. Larrey D, Lohse AW, de Ledinghen V, et al. Rapid and strong antiviral activity of the non-nucleosidic NS5B polymerase inhibitor BI 207127 in combination with peginterferon alfa 2a and ribavirin. J Hepatol 2012;57:39–46.
69. Ray AS, Feng JY, Wang T, et al. 1233 GS-6620: A liver targeted nucleotide prodrug with potent pan-genotype anti-hepatitis C virus activity in vitro. J Hepatol 2011;54:S487.
70. Coelmont L, Hanoulle X, Chatterji U, et al. DEB025 (Alisporivir) inhibits hepatitis C virus replication by preventing a Cyclophilin A induced cis-trans isomerisation in domain II of NS5A. PLoS One 2010;5(10):e13687.

Hepatitis C Virus Viral Assays in the Direct-Acting Antiviral Era

John M. Vierling, MD

KEYWORDS

- Hepatitis C virus • Polymerase chain reaction • Lower limit of quantification
- Limit of detection • Target not detected • Genotype
- Resistance-associated variants • Interleukin 28B

KEY POINTS

- In the direct-acting antiviral (DAA) era of antiviral therapy for Hepatitis C virus (HCV) infections, clinicians must be able to order and interpret results of viral assays for HCV RNA, genotype and subtype, interleukin (IL)-28B genotypes and resistance-associated variants (RAVs).
- Only quantitative assays of HCV RNA with a limit of detection (LOD) of at least 10 to 15 IU/mL are appropriate for managing patients treated with DAA regimens.
- Adherence to stopping rules based on the quantity of HCV RNA at prespecified time points during therapy is mandatory to limit replication of RAVs.
- Eligibility for shorter durations of current DAA therapy requires HCV RNA results of "less than lower limit of quantification (LLOQ), not detected" at prespecified time points during therapy.
- Sustained virologic response (SVR) rates with current DAA therapies are higher for patients with HCV RNA results of "less than LLOQ, not detected" than those of patients with results of "less than LLOQ, detected."
- SVR rates with current DAA therapies are higher in patients with HCV genotype 1b than SVR rates in patients with HCV genotype 1a infections.
- IL-28B genotype remains predictive of SVR using current DAA regimens, but may become less useful with the advent of future regimens.

INTRODUCTION

Approximately 200 million people have chronic hepatitis C virus (HCV) infection worldwide, and clinical sequelae include progression to cirrhosis, liver failure, and development of hepatocellular carcinoma,[1] all of which are increasing in prevalence.[2] As

Author's Disclosures Relevant to this Manuscript: Research grant support and scientific advisory boards for: Abbott, Roche, Vertex, Merck.
Departments of Medicine and Surgery, Liver Center, Baylor College of Medicine and St. Luke's Episcopal Hospital, 6620 Main Street, Suite 1425, Houston, TX 77030, USA
E-mail address: vierling@bcm.edu

a result, cirrhosis, often with hepatocellular carcinoma, due to chronic HCV infection is the primary indication for orthotopic liver transplantation (OLT).[3] Even after successful OLT, recurrent HCV infection in the allograft increases morbidity and mortality.[3,4] There are 6 major genotypes of HCV, and the frequency of these genotypes varies geographically.[1] Most patients with chronic HCV infection in the Americas, Europe, and Japan have genotype 1 infections. However, only approximately 40% of patients infected with HCV genotype 1 (G1) can be cured with pegylated interferon and ribavirin (P/R) antiviral therapy.[5] Thus, development of new therapies with direct-acting antiviral (DAA) agents has concentrated on HCV G1 infections in treatment-naïve[6,7] and treatment experienced patients who previously failed prior therapy with P/R.[8,9]

In 2012, regulatory approvals were granted for DAA HCV NS3/4A HCV protease inhibitors boceprevir (BOC)[10] and telaprevir (TVR)[11] in combination with P/R, launching a new era for DAA treatment of HCV G1 infections. Regimens of BOC/P/R or TVR/P/R achieved SVR rates of 59% to 83%, compared with rates of 15% to 40% in control patients treated with placebo/P/R.[6-9] Conduct of the phase 2 and 3 clinical trials of BOC/P/R and TVR/P/R therapy required accurate quantification of HCV RNA levels at prespecified time points for decisions regarding shortening or extending treatment (response-guided therapy, RGT) or stopping therapy due to futility.[6-9] Futility is defined as both absence of the prospect for SVR and the risk of progressive stimulation of the replication of RAVs[12] in the existing HCV quasispecies.[6-9]

Clinicians using DAA therapies must be familiar with the performance characteristics of commercially available polymerase chain reaction (PCR) assays and appreciate the clinical applications of the of terms used to report results of HCV RNA assays to treat patients with HCV G1 infections.[13] Specifically, clinicians must become adept in the interpretation of HCV RNA assay results to make accurate decisions regarding RGT, apply stopping rules for futility, and to define end-of-treatment response (EOT) and SVR, using DAA regimens. Such knowledge is crucial to maximizing SVR rates, while preventing inappropriate continuation of therapy without the prospect of SVR and its associated risks of adverse events, replication RAVs, and increased costs.[14]

PCR TERMINOLOGY AND DEFINITIONS OF TERMS USED IN HCV RNA PCR ASSAYS

Table 1 defines terms used to describe the analytic performance of HCV RNA viral load assays, commonly used synonyms, and key clinical interpretations.[13,15] **Fig. 1** illustrates the response of plasma HCV RNA to antiviral therapy in a patient with chronic HCV infection. For all quantitative HCV RNA PCR assays, there is a linear range of HCV with defined upper and lower limits of quantification, abbreviated as ULOQ and LLOQ, respectively. HCV RNA amounts greater than ULOQ are reported as ">ULOQ, detected." LLOQ (sometimes abbreviated LLQ) is defined as the lowest concentration of HCV RNA that is both linear and can be accurately quantitated in international units per milliliter of either plasma (preferred because of greater sensitivity of HCV RNA detection) or serum. Thus, LLOQ represents the lowest amount of HCV RNA that is both detectable and quantifiable. The limit of detection (LOD), also referred to as lower limit of detection (LLOD) is defined as the lowest amount of HCV RNA that can be detected with 95% confidence determined using PROBIT regression analysis of the results of repetitive testing of serial dilutions of World Health Organization (WHO) standards added to normal human plasma. Using this definition, it is evident that a given concentration of HCV RNA that is less than LOD may still be reported as "<LLOQ, detected" with a frequency of no more than 5%. Thus, LOD does not define an absolute limit of detection, and HCV RNA can be detected below this value. As the actual amount of HCV RNA approaches 1 IU/mL, the ability to detect

Table 1
Performance terminology, definitions, synonyms and interpretations of using quantitative HCV RNA PCR assays

Performance Terms	Definition	Synonyms	Interpretation
ULOQ	Highest concentration of analyte that is both linear and accurate Units: IU/mL	None	Highest level of HCV RNA that can be accurately detected and quantified
LLOQ[1]	Lowest concentration of analyte that is both linear and accurate Units: IU/mL	LOQ	Lowest level of HCV RNA that can be accurately detected and quantified
LOD	Lowest concentration of analyte that can be detected with rate of ≥95% based on PROBIT regression analysis of serially diluted controls Always ≤LLOQ	LLOD	Detectable, but not quantifiable, HCV RNA Clinically significant
<LLOQ, detected	Analyte detectable but not quantifiable Always <LLOQ, but only 95% of values lie between LLOQ and LOD, since 5% can be below LOD	Detectable or BLOQ, detected	HCV RNA detectable Clinically significant
<LLOQ, not detected	Analyte detectable but not quantifiable Always <LLOQ, but only 95% of values lie between LLOQ and LOD, since 5% can be below LOD	Undetectable or BLOD	HCV RNA not detectable Clinically significant
TND	No amplification of analyte Approaches or equals: 0 IU/mL	Undetectable or BLOD	Only valid definition of undetectable HCV RNA Clinically significant

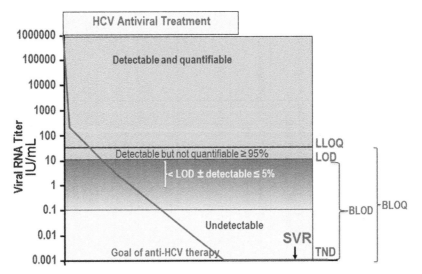

Fig. 1. Interpretation of virologic response of HCV RNA during antiviral therapy. (*Courtesy of JM Vierling, MD, Houston, TX. Presented at The Combination and Novel HCV Therapies Conference 2012.*)

it rapidly decreases (see **Fig. 1**). The term "target not detected" (TND) is applicable when the concentration of analyte approximates 0 IU/mL. Thus, TND is truly synonymous with undetectable. Most laboratories report results of "<LLOQ, not detected," while a minority may report "undetectable" or TND (see **Table 1**). In a recent publication, the US Food and Drug Administration (FDA) introduced new terms of below limit of quantification (BLOQ) for less than LLOQ and below limit of detection (BLOD) to encompass both less than LOD and TND (see **Table 1** and **Fig. 1**).[16] They also used the term undetectable as a synonym for results reported as either "<LLOQ, not detected" or "TND". It is unlikely that these new terms will replace recommendations for standardization of reports of PCR results.[15]

Using these definitions, the clinician can accurately interpret results of HCV RNA PCR assays. For values exceeding the ULOQ, results may be reported as greater than ULOQ or as ">ULOQ, detected." Results that are in the linear quantifiable range between the ULOQ and LLOQ, the report states the quantity of HCV RNA in international units per milliliter. For results of HCV RNA less than LLOQ, the report will indicate the actual value of the LLOQ for the specific PCR assay in international units per milliliter. In addition, results less than LLOQ will also state whether HCV RNA was detected or not detected. A result of "<LLOQ, detected" indicates that HCV RNA is either detectable between the LOD and the LLOQ (expected in ≥95% of instances) or below both the LLOQ and the LOD (expected in ≤5% of instances). Conversely, a result of "<LLOQ, not detected" indicates that HCV RNA is <LOD or not present (TND) or ≤1 IU/mL (see **Fig. 1**).

QUALITATIVE AND QUANTITATIVE HCV RNA ASSAYS

Table 2 summarizes the performance characteristics of qualitative and quantitative HCV RNA assays using pangenotypic LOD values. Among qualitative assays, several have sufficient sensitivity (≤10 IU/mL) to be considered useful for assessment of the response to DAA-based therapies. However, the absence of quantitative results precludes their use for monitoring of patients for determination of either stopping rules for futility or eligibility for RGT. Thus, DAA therapies currently require use of quantitative HCV RNA PCR assays or assays that apply a qualitative assay to specimens with HCV RNA levels less than LLOQ (see **Table 2**).

QUANTITATIVE HCV RNA PCR ASSAYS FOR HCV GENOTYPE 1 INFECTIONS

Table 3 compares the performance characteristics of the 6 major quantitative HCV PCR assays available for the monitoring and treatment of HCV G1 infections in the United States. The COBAS TaqMan HCV Test, v2.0 for use with High Pure System (Roche Molecular Systems, Pleasanton, CA) is the assay used in both the BOC/P/R and TVR/P/R registration trials with an approved LLOQ of 25 IU/mL and LOD of 10 to 15 IU/mL.[10,11,13] However, the LOD for HCV G1 in the BOC/P/R and TVR/P/R trials was independently determined by the reference laboratories, resulting in an LOD of 9.3 IU/mL for the phase 2 and 3 trials of BOC/P/R[6,8,17] and 10 IU/mL for the phase 2 and 3 TVR/P/R trials.[7,9,18] Although this PCR assay is commercially available, many clinical laboratories prefer the COBAS AmpliPrep/COBAS TaqMan HCV Test because of its simplicity. This assay has an LLOQ of 43 IU/mL and LOD for HCV G1 of 7.1 IU/mL. The recently FDA-approved Abbott RealTime HCV (Abbott Molecular Inc, Des Plaines, IL) assay has an LLOQ of 12 IU/mL and an LOD of 10.5 IU/mL for HCV G1. It is noteworthy that the pan-genotypic analysis of the Abbott RealTime HCV RNA assay found the LLOQ and LOD to be identical. However, clinicians receiving reports using this assay for patients with HCV G1 infection will encounter results of "<LLOQ, detected" and "<LLOQ, not detected," because the LOD for HCV G1 is less than LLOQ. The HEPTIMAX (Quest Diagnostics, Madison, NJ) assay screens with the COBAS AmpliPrep/COBAS TaqMan HCV Test and retests samples with <43 IU/mL using the transcription-mediated amplification (TMA) method. The analytical performance characteristics were determined by Quest Diagnostics Nichols Institute as LLOQ of 5 IU/mL and LOD of 0.7 IU/mL. The performance characteristics for QuantaSure and QuantaSure Plus (LabCorp, Burlington, NC) are also robust. The LLOQ and LOD are both 2 IU/mL for QuantaSure. For QuantaSure Plus, the LLOQ is 10 IU/mL, and the LOD is 2 IU/mL. The availability of these more sensitive, quantitative HCV RNA assays raises the question of clinical meaning of detecting quantifiable HCV RNA at concentrations of between 2 and 9 IU/mL, when these would have been regarded as "<LLOQ, not detected" on current DAA therapy based on the LOD of 9.3 IU/mL in the BOC/P/R[6,8] and the LOD of 10 IU/mL in the TVR/P/R[7,9] trials. Such patients are at theoretic risk of relapse,[19,20] but a recent report indicated a high probability of SVR.[21]

LOD VARIES FOR HCV GENOTYPES

Table 4 illustrates differences in LOD calculated using PROBIT regression analyses of panels of different HCV genotypes in studies of the Abbott RealTime HCV assay.[22] LOD varied substantially among the major genotypes. Thus, clinicians must inquire about the LOD of an assay for a particular genotype and not rely on the LOD representing a pan–genotypic average. As noted in **Table 3**, the LOD for HCV G1 tends to be lower than the LOD based on a pan-genotypic average.

CLINICAL SIGNIFICANCE OF RESULTS "<LLOQ, DETECTED" VERSUS "<LLOQ, NOT DETECTED"

Harrington and colleagues[16] at the FDA analyzed the proportion of subjects with HCV RNA levels "<LLOQ, detected" versus "<LLOQ, not detected" in selected phase 2 and

Table 2
Performance characteristics and uses of qualitative and quantitative HCV RNA PCR assays

Assay	Method	Quantitative Range LLOQ-ULOQ	LOD IU/mL (Plasma)	Clinical Use
Amplicor HCV v1.0	Manual Reverse transcriptase-PCR	Qualitative Only	50	Diagnosis and monitoring
COBAS Amplicor HCV v2.0	(RT-PCR) Semiautomated RT-PCR	Qualitative Only	50	Diagnosis and monitoring
Ampliscreen	Semiautomated RT-PCR	Qualitative Only	<50	Blood screening
Versant HCV RNA Qualitative Assay	Semiautomated TMA	Qualitative Only	9.6	Diagnosis and monitoring
Procleix HIV-1/HCV Assay	Manual TMA	Qualitative Only	50	Blood screening
Amplicor HCV Monitor	Manual RT-PCR	Quantitative 600–500,000	N/A	LOD not suitable for DAA therapy
COBAS Amplicor HCV Monitor V2.0	Semiautomated RT-PCR	Quantitative 600–500,000	600	LOD not suitable for DAA therapy
Artus HCV QS-RGQ Assay	Semiautomated-PCR	Quantitative 67.6–17,700,00	36.2	LOD not suitable for DAA therapy
Versant HCV RNA 3.0 Assay (bDNA)	Semiautomated bDNA signal amplification	Quantitative 615–700,000	615	LOD not suitable for DAA therapy

LCx HCV RNA-Quantitative Assay	Semiautomated RT-PCR	Quantitative 25–2,630,000	23	LOD not suitable for DAA therapy
QuantaSure	Semiautomated RT-PCR	Quantitative 2–2,000,000	2	LOD suitable for DAA therapy
QuantaSure Plus	Automated RT-PCR	Quantitative 10–100,000,000	10	LOD suitable for DAA therapy
COBAS TaqMan HCV Test	Semiautomated RT-PCR	Quantitative 43–69,000,000	18 overall 7.1 G1a/1b	LOD for G1 suitable for antiviral therapy
COBAS TaqMan HCV Test v2.0 for use with High Pure System	Semiautomated RT-PCR	Quantitative 25–300,000,000	15	LOD for G1 suitable for antiviral therapy
Abbott RealTime HCV Assay	Semiautomated RT-PCR	Quantitative 12–100,000,000	12	LOD for G1 suitable for antiviral therapy
HEPTIMAX	Two-Step Test: – COBAS TaqMan HCV Test Semiautomated RT PCR – Followed by Quantitative Bayer TMA for samples with results <43 IU/mL	Quantitative Step 1 43–69,000,000 Step 2 5–7000 Overall: 5–69,000,000	5	LOD for G1 suitable for antiviral therapy

Abbreviation: TMA, transmission-mediated amplification.

Table 3
Comparison of HCV RNA PCR assays for HCV genotype 1

HCV PCR Assay (Manufacturer)	LLOQ	LOD (Plasma) Genotype 1
COBAS TaqMan HCV Test v2.0 for use with High Pure System	25 IU/mL	9.3–10 IU/mL
COBAS TaqMan HCV Test	43 IU/mL	7.1 IU/mL
Abbott RealTime HCV Assay	12 IU/mL	10.5 IU/mL
HEPTIMAX	5 IU/mL	5 IU/mL
QuantaSure	2 IU/mL	2 IU/mL
QuantaSure Plus	10 IU/mL	2 IU/mL

phase 3 clinical trials of BOC/P/R and TVR/PR between 2 and 24 weeks of treatment. Their analysis showed that results of "<LLOQ, detected" were frequent in both trials (**Fig. 2**). In the BOC/P/R phase 3 trial in treatment-naïve patients (Serine Protease Inhibitor Trial [SPRINT-2]),[6] 52% of all subjects had at least 1 result of "<LLOQ, detected," while in the TVR/P/R phase 3 trial in treatment experienced patients (REALIZE),[9] 67% of patients had at least 1 result reported as "<LLOQ, detected." Of note, the proportion of patients with these results peaked before or near to prespecified time points used for decisions about RGT (week 8 for BOC/P/R and week 4 for TVR/P/R without a lead in). In the single arm of the TVR/P/R trial for treatment-experienced patients that included a 4-week P/R lead in, the peak frequency of results "<LLOQ, detected" was postponed by 2 to 4 weeks.[9]

The most important clinical finding of Harrington and colleagues[16] was that subjects with results of "<LLOQ, detected" had reduced SVR rates compared with subjects with results of "<LLOQ, not detected" at similar time points during therapy with either BOC/P/R or TVR/P/R (**Fig. 3**). Subjects with reports of "<LLOQ, detected" at the key RGT time points of week 8 for BOC or week 4 for TVR, SVR rates were approximately 20% lower than those of subjects with results of "<LLOQ, not detected." In the TVR/P/R trial for treatment-naïve subjects,[7] differences in SVR rates were less pronounced, but the same trend was identified. Importantly, both phase 2 trials of BOC/P/R and TVR/P/R showed that subjects benefitted from extended therapy if they had results of "<LLOQ, detected" at key RGT time points. SVR rates were also lower among subjects who transitioned from "<LLOQ, detected" to "<LLOQ, not detected" during therapy with BOC/P/R compared with those of subjects who achieved "<LLOLQ, not detected" at an earlier time point (**Fig. 4**). The SVR rates in patients randomized to RGT using BOC/P/R therapy who had "<LLOQ, detected" versus "<LLOQ, not detected" could not be studied, since only subjects with results of "<LLOQ, not detected" at key decision time points were eligible for RGT. The results of the FDA''s post hoc analysis underscores the importance of differentiating between results of "<LLOQ, detected" versus "<LLOQ, not detected" when using either BOC/P/R or TVR/P/R DAA therapies.

Table 4
Example of variability of limit of detection for different HCV genotypes

HCV PCR Assay	G1	G2	G3	G4	G5	G6
COBAS TaqMan HCV Test	7.1 IU/mL	15.3 IU/mL	9.8 IU/mL	5.6 IU/mL	18.3 IU/mL	9.7 IU/mL
Abbott RealTime HCV Assay	8.3 IU/mL	6.4 IU/mL	6.6 IU/mL	11.0 IU/mL	6.7 IU/mL	4.4 IU/mL

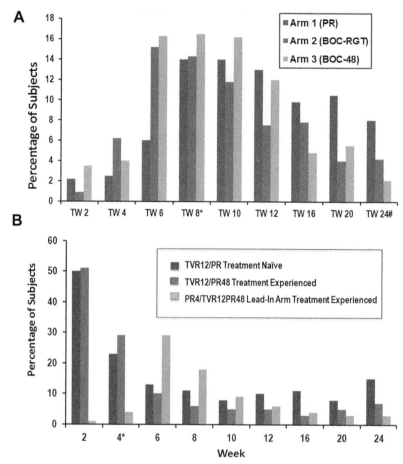

Fig. 2. Frequency of HCV RNA PCR results of "<LLOQ, detected" at key time points on therapy during the registration trials of (*A*) boceprevir in treatment-naïve patients (SPRINT-2) and (*B*) telaprevir in treatment-naïve (ADVANCE) and treatment-experienced patients (REALIZE). *Abbreviations:* BOC, boceprevir; BOC-48, 48 week treatment arm; PR, pegylated interferon and ribavirin; PR4/TVR12/PR, arm with 4 weeks PR lead-in before adding TVR in REALIZE trial; RGT, response-guided therapy; TW, treatment week; TVR, telaprevir. (*Courtesy of* JM Vierling, MD, Houston, TX. Presented at The Combination and Novel HCV Therapies Conference 2012.)

DEFINITIONS OF EOT AND SVR IN THE DAA ERA

Using BOC/P/R or TVR/P/R regimens, a successful EOT response should be defined as an HCV RNA of "<LLOQ, not detected" using an assay with an LOD of less than or equal to 10 to −15 IU/mL.[10,11,23,24] This is supported by evidence that an EOT HCV RNA "<LLOQ, detected" results in a lower SVR rate.[16] Using P/R therapy without a DAA, SVR was defined as an undetectable HCV RNA level greater than or equal to 24 weeks after treatment using a PCR assay with an LLOQ of ≤50 IU/mL. In contrast, the FDA defined SVR in the package inserts for both BOC/P/R and TVR/P/R therapies as <25 IU/mL, which is less than LLOQ of the COBAS TaqMan HCV Test, v2.0 for use with High Pure System used in phase 3 trials of both DAA regimens.[23,24] Since virtually all relapses occur by post-treatment week 12, results of

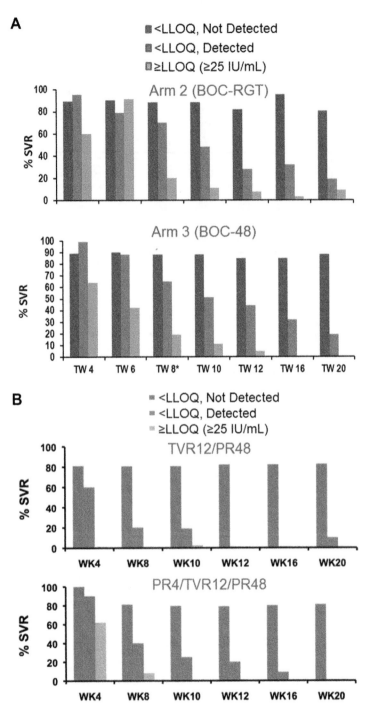

Fig. 3. Differences in SVR rates in patients with HCV RNA PCR results of "<LLOQ, not detected" versus "<LLOQ, detected" at key time points on therapy during the registration trials of (*A*) boceprevir in treatment-naïve patients (SPRINT-2) and (*B*) telaprevir in treatment-naïve (ADVANCE) and treatment-experienced patients (REALIZE). *Abbreviations*: BOC, boceprevir; BOC-48, 48-week treatment arm; PR, pegylated interferon and ribavirin; PR4/TVR12/PR, arm with 4 weeks PR lead-in before adding TVR in REALIZE trial; RGT, response-guided therapy; SVR, sustained virologic response; TW, treatment week; TVR, telaprevir. (*Courtesy of* JM Vierling, MD, Houston, TX. Presented at The Combination and Novel HCV Therapies Conference 2012.)

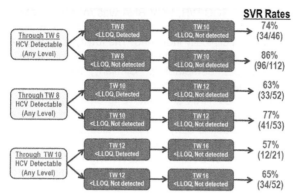

Fig. 4. Differences in SVR rates in patients whose HCV RNA PCR results transitioned from "<LLOQ, detected" to "<LLOQ, not detected" during the phase 3 trial of boceprevir in treatment-naïve patients (SPRINT-2). *Abbreviations:* SVR, sustained virologic response; TW, treatment week. (*Courtesy of* JM Vierling, MD, Houston, TX. Presented at The Combination and Novel HCV Therapies Conference 2012.)

less than LLOQ at week 24 are now deemed sufficient to define SVR using DAA regimens.[25] In clinical practice (see **Table 3**), SVR for BOC/P/R and TVR/P/R DAA regimens is still defined as HCV RNA less than <LLOQ, 24 or more weeks after therapy using commercially available assays. However, the LLOQ level of 25 IU/mL only applies to the COBAS TaqMan HCV Test, v2.0 for use with High Pure System used in phase 3 trials of BOC/P/R and TVR/P/R. Currently available HCV RNA assays have LLOQs that vary from 2 to 43 IU/mL (see **Table 3**).

ELIGIBILITY FOR RGT

Decisions to shorten therapy in the phase 3 BOC/P/R and TVR/P/R trials for treatment-naïve and treatment-experienced patients was have been based on declines of HCV RNA levels at prespecified time points to values of "<LLOQ, not detected".[6–9,16] As noted previously, patients with results of "<LLOQ, detected" at these key time points benefitted from extended therapy.[16] Patients eligible for RGT using BOC/P/R include those who are noncirrhotic, treatment-naïve patients, and treatment-experienced patients with prior relapse or partial response.[12,23] The criterion is a sustained HCV RNA level "<LLOQ, not detected" from week 8 (ie, week 4 of combination BOC/P/R therapy after a 4- week lead-in with P/R) through week 24. Patients eligible for RGT with TVR/P/R include non–cirrhotic, treatment-naïve patients and previous relapsers among treatment-experienced patients.[24] The criterion for RGT is a sustained HCV level "<LLOQ, not detected" from week 4 of TVR/P/R therapy through week 12.

STOPPING RULES FOR FUTILITY

Failure to achieve HCV RNA on-treatment levels of "<LLOQ, not detected" not only impacts decisions regarding RGT and diminishes SVR rates, but also results in selection and uninhibited replication of RAVs within the pretreatment HCV quasispecies.[12,26,27] To prevent continuation of therapy that would ultimately not achieve SVR with either BOC/P/R or TVR/P/R, specific stopping rules were incorporated in the phase 3 trial designs.[28,29]

For the phase 3 trials of BOC/P/R, HCV RNA was monitored at week 4 (end of 4 week P/R lead-in), week 8 (week 4 of combination therapy with BOC/P/R), and weeks 12 and 24, as well as when clinically indicated. The futility stopping rule for the trial in treatment-naïve patients was detectable HCV RNA at week 24 (ie, greater than or equal to LLOQ or "<LLOQ, detectable").[6] Similarly, the futility stopping rule for treatment-experienced patients with prior relapse or partial response after P/R therapy was detectable HCV RNA at week 12 (greater than or equal to LLOQ or "<LLOQ, detectable").[8] Jacobson and colleagues[28] analyzed retrospectively both phase 3 BOC/P/R trials to define early stopping rules based on the hypothesis that specific HCV RNA levels could be identified that would minimize the risk of continuing therapy without a prospect of SVR, while preventing premature discontinuation of therapy for those with a prospect of achieving SVR. Specifically, they assessed the impact of different stopping rules using cutoff values greater than or equal to LOD, greater than or equal to LLOQ or ≥ 50, ≥ 100, or ≥ 1000 IU/mL or $<2 \log_{10}$ and $<3 \log_{10}$ declines from baseline at week 8 or week 12 for treatment-naïve patients or week 16 for prior relapsers or partial responders. For treatment-naïve patients, a stopping rule of HCV RNA ≥ 100 IU/mL at week 12 (week 8 of combination BOC/P/R therapy), would have discontinued therapy in 65 of 195 patients without sacrificing the potential for SVR in any patient (sensitivity 33%, specificity 100%). Among treatment-experienced patients with relapse or partial response, 5 of 6 patients who had HCV RNA levels at week 12 of "<LLOQ, detected" achieved SVR, despite meeting a futility stopping rule. An additional patient with a week 12 HCV RNA level of 148 IU/mL also continued therapy and achieved SVR. Overall, the data indicated that a stopping rule of HCV RNA of ≥ 100 IU/mL at week 12 was highly predictive of failure to achieve SVR in both treatment-naïve and treatment-experienced patients. An HCV RNA level of ≥ 100 IU/mL at week 12 constituted a stopping rule for futility, as did a confirmed HCV RNA level of greater than or equal to LLOQ or "<LLOQ, detected" at week 24. These combined stopping rules afforded patients the benefit of early discontinuation in the absence of the prospect of an SVR, while minimizing the risk of prematurely discontinuing therapy when there was a prospect of achieving SVR.

In TVR/P/R trials, HCV RNA was monitored at weeks 4 and 12 of TVR/P/R therapy. HCV RNA levels of >1000 IU/mL at either week 4 or 12 constituted stopping rules.[7,9] In addition, HCV RNA greater than or equal to LLOQ or "<LLOQ, detected" at week 24 was grounds for discontinuation of the P/R extension of therapy. Adda and colleagues[29] retrospectively analyzed the performance characteristics of the TVR stopping rules for futility in the phase 3 trials of TVR/P/R therapy. HCV RNA levels >1000 IU/mL at week 4 were identified in 1.7% (14 of 844) of treatment-naïve patients, 0.7% (1 of 138) of prior relapsers, 0% (0 of 46) of prior partial responders and 14% (10 of 70) of prior null responders. Among the 25 total patients with HCV RNA levels >1000 IU/mL (n = 14 treatment-naïve, n = 11 treatment-experienced), none achieved SVR with continued treatment. Analyses of HCV RNA levels at week 2 showed that 92% (23 of 25) of patients who had HCV RNA levels >1000 IU/mL at week 4 had lower levels of HCV RNA at week 2, indicating the week 4 levels of >1000 IU/mL represented a rebound from an earlier nadir.

Despite clear evidence-based stopping rules for futility using either BOC/P/R or TVR/P/R therapies, patients are often incredulous and adversarial when admonished to discontinue therapy because of viral loads of ≥ 100 IU/mL for BOC/P/R regimens or >1000 IU/mL for TVR/P/R regimens. Most patients view either of these HCV RNA levels as evidence of an extraordinary decline from baseline HCV RNA levels, and disbelieve that they represent failure to respond to the DAA regimen. It is important that clinicians be well informed about the details of the analyses of the stopping rules that definitively support discontinuation of therapy for futility in both treatment-naïve and treatment-experienced populations. It is also important to explain the importance of avoiding unnecessary exposure to continued therapy without the prospect of SVR because of the risk of stimulating replication of RAVs.

HCV GENOTYPING

There are 6 major HCV genotypes that vary in proportions geographically (**Fig. 5**).[1] In the United States, approximately 75% of patients are infected with HCV G1, which has 2 subtypes: 1a and 1b. In the United States, approximately 67% of patients with HCV infection have G1a subtype, and 33% have G1b subtype, while the proportion of patients with G1b in Europe and Japan is substantially greater. HCV genotyping assays (**Table 5**) are readily available, and all patients with HCV infection must be genotyped for discussion of therapeutic options. Incorrect typing among major genotypes occurs in less than 3% of patients; a small minority of patients has either an indeterminate result or is infected with more than 1 genotype. In the phase 3 clinical trials of BOC/P/R[6,8] and TVR/P/R[7,9] therapies for HCV G1 patients, rates of SVR were appreciably higher in patients infected with G1b than those infected with G1a (**Fig. 6**). It is hoped that newer DAA therapies will negate the disparity in SVR rates between HCV G1a and G1b infections.

HCV RESISTANCE-ASSOCIATED VARIANTS

HCV within the quasispecies, referred to as RAV, exhibits amino acid substitutions in the NS3 serine protease that confer resistance to either BOC or TVR.[12,26,27,30,31] RAVs are present within the pretreatment HCV quasispecies in up to 7% of patients before treatment.[31] RAVs have a selective advantage for replication when the combined antiviral effects of the BOC/P/R or TVR/P/R are insufficient to terminate HCV replication. The risk of enhancing replication of RAVs also increases if patients fail to take all 3 drugs or miss doses of either BOC or TVR. To minimize the emergence of RAVs from the quasispecies requires patient compliance with the treatment regimen and strict adherence to stopping rules for futility. RAVs are relatively less fit than wild-type HCV, and do not appear to worsen liver disease. Serial studies have shown that the proportions of all known RAVs decline within the quasispecies after

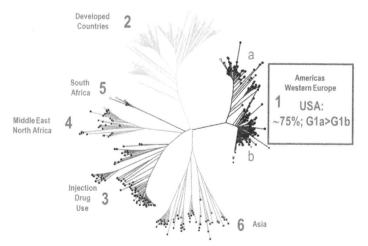

Fig. 5. The phylogeny of the 6 major HCV genotypes. (*Courtesy of* JM Vierling, MD, Houston, TX. Presented at The Combination and Novel HCV Therapies Conference 2012.)

Table 5	
HCV genotyping assays	
Genotype Assay (Manufacturer)	**Method**
Trugene 5' NC HCV Genotyping Kit	Direct sequence analysis of the 5' noncoding region
INNO-LiPa HCV II	Reverse hybridization analysis using genotype-specific oligonucleotide probes located in the 5' noncoding region
Versant HCV Genotyping Assay 2.0	Reverse hybridization analysis using genotype-specific oligonucleotide probes located in the 5' noncoding region
Abbott RealTime HCV Genotype II	Genotype-specific real-time PCR of the 5' noncoding region and NS5B

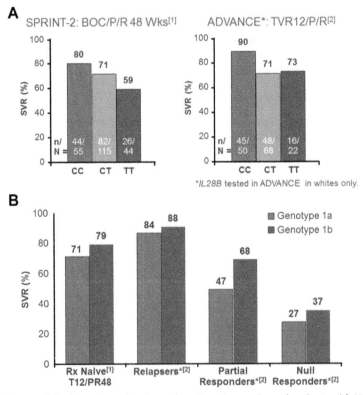

Fig. 6. SVR rates differ in treatment-naïve and treatment-experienced patients with HCV genotype 1a versus genotype 1b using (A) boceprevir or (B) telaprevir DAA regimens. *Abbreviations*: BOC, boceprevir; PR, pegylated interferon and ribavirin; Rx, treatment; RGT, response-guided therapy; SVR, sustained virologic response. (*Courtesy of* JM Vierling, MD, Houston, TX. Presented at The Combination and Novel HCV Therapies Conference 2012. Data from [A] Jacobson IM, McHutchison JG, Dusheiko G, et al. Telaprevir for previously untreated chronic hepatitis C virus infection. N Engl J Med 2011;364:2405–16; Zeuzem S, Andreone P, Pol S, et al. REALIZE trial final results: telaprevir-based regimen for genotype 1 hepatitis C virus infection in patients with prior null response, partial response or relapse to peginterferon/ribavirin. J Hepatol 2011;54:S3; [B] Poordad F, McCone Jr J, Bacon BR, et al. Boceprevir for untreated chronic HCV genotype 1 infection. N Engl J Med 2011;364:1195–206; Bacon BR, Gordon SC, Lawitz E, et al. Boceprevir for previously treated chronic HCV genotype 1 infection. N Engl J Med 2011;364:1207–17.)

withdrawal of either BOC/P/R or TVR/P/R. However, specific RAVs remain detectable with population sequencing, which has thresholds of detection ranging from 20% to 25% for specific RAVs, for up to 2.5 years.[27] Genotype 1a has a lower genetic barrier to resistance than genotype 1b due to the fact that genotype 1a requires single nucleotide substitutions to generate changes in the amino acids at specific sites, while genotype 1b requires sequential nucleotide substitutions to generate the same amino acid replacements.[26,32,33] The frequency of RAVs with specific amino acid substitutions differs between G1a and G1b, but are identical for both BOC and TVR.[26]

A commercial assay, HCV GenoSure NS3/4A (Monogram Biosciences, South San Francisco, CA), is now available to detect RAVs with a maximum sensitivity for detection of an individual RAV of 10%.[34] However, the clinical utility remains unclear, since RAVs are uniformly present whenever patients meet stopping rules for futility or develop on-treatment virologic breakthrough. In the future, as is true in human immunodeficiency virus (HIV) infection, it is conceivable that the HCV RAV profile of patients who failed BOC/P/R, TVR/P/R, or future DAA therapies may aid in the selection of specific DAA regimens without cross-resistance.

IL-28B SINGLE NUCLEOTIDE POLYMORPHISMS IN THE DAA ERA

The ability to comprehensively screen the entire human genome with a genome-wide association study (GWAS) led to the discovery of the strong association between IL-28B single nucleotide polymorphisms (SNPs) and the response of HCV G1 patients to treatment with P/R.[35,36] Subsequent GWAS analysis showed that SNPs strongly predictive of SVR in HCV G1 patients treated with P/R were less common in patients with chronic HCV infection than in healthy controls. This discrepancy was explained by the fact that the same IL-28B SNPs that predicted response to P/R in chronically infected patients were significantly associated with spontaneous clearance of acute HCV infection.[37]

The predictive IL-28B SNPs, rs12979860 and rs8099917, lie within a haplotype block on chromosome 19 that codes for interferon-lamda-3 (IFN-λ3).[36] In most populations, these 2 SNPs are equally informative, because they are inherited together as a result of strong linkage disequilibrium. In contrast, in African Americans, the SNP rs12979860 is more closely associated with SVR with P/R therapy than is the SNP rs8099917.[36] With the SNP rs12979860, SVR rates with P/R therapy for HCV G1 infections are highest for patients with genotype CC, intermediate for heterozygous CT, and lowest for those with genotype TT. For the SNP rs8099917, the SVR rates with P/R therapy are greatest for the TT genotype, intermediate for the GT genotype, and least for the GG genotype. The frequency of the good response CC allele varies according to race and ethnic background, with a hierarchy of Asian > Caucasian > Latino > African.[36] The IL-28B genotype explains much, but not all, of the differences in SVR rates observed with P/R therapy for HCV G1 infections in different racial and ethnic populations. A similar association also exists between IL-28B genotype and SVR after P/R therapy of patients with HCV G1-HIV coinfections.[38] IL-28B genotype is also related to treatment outcomes in patients with recurrent HCV G1 infections in allografts after orthotopic liver transplantation, but in this chimeric situation, IL-28B alleles of both the recipient and donor liver play roles in the risk of progression of recurrent HCV infection and the potential for SVR with P/R therapy.[39–46]

The value of IL-28B genotyping to predict SVR is greatest for P/R treatment of HCV G1 infection, but it also remains predictive for SVR using either BOC/P/R or TVR/P/R regimens in treatment-naïve or treatment-experienced patients (**Fig. 7**).[6–9] The predictive utility for IL-28B genotypes extends to HCV G4 infections, but is less predictive for SVR in HCV G2 or G3 infections.[36] In HCV G2 and G3 infections, the favorable CC genotype correlates with early, rapid virologic kinetics, but does not correlate with SVR.

The clinical use of commercially available testing for the IL-28B genotypes for the SNP rs12979860 in the DAA era is not completely characterized, but some facts provide guidance. First, the IL-28B genotype is predictive of SVR for both treatment-naïve and treatment-experienced patients with HCV G1 infections, whether treated with P/R alone or either BOC/P/R or TVR/P/R. Second, it is also predictive of SVR in patients with HCV G4 infections treated with P/R. Third, IL-28B genotyping has no predictive value for SVR in HCV G2 or G3 infections and cannot be recommended. It is likely that future therapies of DAAs with higher barriers to HCV resistance combined with P/R will achieve higher rates of SVR, lessening the clinical utility of IL-28B genotype testing before therapy. If interferon-free DAA regimens are successful, IL-28B genotype testing may no longer be clinically useful, unless it were predictive of the patient's endogenous interferon responses during therapy.

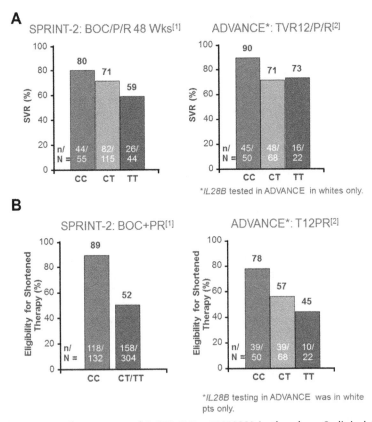

Fig. 7. SVR rates and genotypes of IL-28B SNP rs12979860 in the phase 3 clinical trials of boceprevir or telaprevir therapy for treatment-naïve patients. *Abbreviations:* BOC, boceprevir; PR, pegylated interferon and ribavirin; SVR, sustained virologic response; Wks, weeks. (*Courtesy of* JM Vierling, MD, Houston, TX. Presented at The Combination and Novel HCV Therapies Conference 2012.)

REFERENCES

1. Bostan N, Mahmood T. An overview about hepatitis C: a devastating virus. Crit Rev Microbiol 2010;36:91–133.
2. Davis GL, Alter MJ, El-Serag H, et al. Aging of hepatitis C virus (HCV)-infected persons in the United States: a multiple cohort model of HCV prevalence and disease progression. Gastroenterology 2010;138:513–21.
3. Angelico M. Epidemiology and outcome of hepatitis C relapse in transplant recipients. Transplant Proc 2011;43:2457–8.
4. Selzner N, Guindi M, Renner EL, et al. Immune-mediated complications of the graft in interferon-treated hepatitis C positive liver transplant recipients. J Hepatol 2011;55:207–17.
5. McHutchison JG, Lawitz EJ, Shiffman ML, et al. Peginterferon alfa-2b or alfa-2a with ribavirin for treatment of hepatitis C infection. N Engl J Med 2009;361: 580–93.
6. Poordad F, McCone J Jr, Bacon BR, et al. Boceprevir for untreated chronic HCV genotype 1 infection. N Engl J Med 2011;364:1195–206.
7. Jacobson IM, McHutchison JG, Dusheiko G, et al. Telaprevir for previously untreated chronic hepatitis C virus infection. N Engl J Med 2011;364: 2405–16.
8. Bacon BR, Gordon SC, Lawitz E, et al. Boceprevir for previously treated chronic HCV genotype 1 infection. N Engl J Med 2011;364:1207–17.
9. Zeuzem S, Andreone P, Pol S, et al. Telaprevir for retreatment of HCV infection. N Engl J Med 2011;364:2417–28.
10. US Food, Drug Administration. Antiviral drug advisory committee meeting and briefing materials for boceprevir. US Food and Drug Administration; 2011.
11. US Food, Drug Administration. Antiviral drug advisory board meeting and briefing materials for telaprevir. US Food and Drug Administration; 2011.
12. Halfon P, Sarrazin C. Future treatment of chronic hepatitis C with direct acting antivirals: is resistance important? Liver Int 2012;32(Suppl 1):79–87.
13. Cobb B, Pockros PJ, Vilchez RA, et al. HCV RNA viral load assessments in the era of direct acting antivirals. Am J Gastroenterol, in press.
14. Soriano V, Vispo E, Poveda E, et al. Treatment failure with new hepatitis C drugs. Expert Opin Pharmacother 2012;13:313–23.
15. Wedemeyer H, Jensen DM, Godofsky E, et al. Recommendations for standardized nomenclature and definitions of viral response in trials of HCV investigational agents. Hepatology 2012. http://dx.doi.org/10.1002/hep.25888.
16. Harrington PR, Zeng W, Naeger LK. Clinical relevance of detectable but not quantifiable hepatitis C virus RNA during boceprevir or telaprevir treatment. Hepatology 2012;55:1048–57.
17. Kwo PY, Lawitz EJ, McCone J, et al. Efficacy of boceprevir, an NS3 protease inhibitor, in combination with peginterferon alfa-2b and ribavirin in treatment-naive patients with genotype 1 hepatitis C infection (SPRINT-1): an open-label, randomised, multicentre phase 2 trial. Lancet 2010;376:705–16.
18. Burney T, Dusheiko G. Overview of the PROVE studies evaluating the use of telaprevir in chronic hepatitis C genotype 1 patients. Expert Rev Anti Infect Ther 2011;9:151–60.
19. Kadam JS, Gonzalez SA, Ahmed F, et al. Prognostic significance of hepatitis C virus RNA detection by transcription-mediated amplification with negative polymerase chain reaction during therapy with peginterferon alpha and ribavirin. Dig Dis Sci 2007;52:2525–30.

20. Morishima C, Morgan TR, Everhart JE, et al. Interpretation of positive transcription-mediated amplification test results from polymerase chain reaction-negative samples obtained after treatment of chronic hepatitis C. Hepatology 2008;48: 1412–9.

21. Thadani A, Harley J, Rubin J, et al. Clinical significance of discordant positive hepatitis C virus transcription-mediated amplification following end of treatment response. Dig Dis Sci 2012;57:239–42.

22. Abbott Real Time HCV PCR: PMA P100017 FDA summary of safety and effectiveness. 2011.

23. Victrelis (boceprevir) capsules. U.S. prescribing information. Whitehouse Station (NJ): Merck; 2011.

24. Incivek (telaprevir) film coated tablets. US prescribing information. Cambridge (MA): Vertex Pharmaceuticals; 2011.

25. New DAA FDA guidance. Available at: www.natap.org/2012/HCV/041012_03.htm. Accessed August, 2012.

26. Gambarin-Gelwan M, Jacobson IM. Resistance-associated variants in chronic hepatitis C patients treated with protease inhibitors. Curr Gastroenterol Rep 2012;14:47–54.

27. Susser S, Vermehren J, Forestier N, et al. Analysis of long-term persistence of resistance mutations within the hepatitis C virus NS3 protease after treatment with telaprevir or boceprevir. J Clin Virol 2011;52:321–7.

28. Jacobson IM, Marcellin P, Zeuzem S, et al. Refinement of stopping rules during treatment of hepatitis C genotype 1 infection with boceprevir and peginterferon/ribavirin. Hepatology 2012;56:567–75.

29. Adda N, Bartels DJ, Gritz L, et al. Understanding futility rules in telaprevir combination treatment. Clin Gastroenterol Hepatol, in press.

30. Meyer SD, Dierynck I, Ghys A, et al. Characterization of telaprevir treatment outcomes and resistance in patients with prior treatment failure: results from the realize trial. Hepatology 2012. http://dx.doi.org/10.1002/hep.25962.

31. Rong L, Ribeiro RM, Perelson AS. Modeling quasispecies and drug resistance in hepatitis C patients treated with a protease inhibitor. Bull Math Biol 2012;74: 1789–817.

32. Delang L, Vliegen I, Froeyen M, et al. Comparative study of the genetic barriers and pathways towards resistance of selective inhibitors of hepatitis C virus replication. Antimicrob Agents Chemother 2011;55:4103–13.

33. Imhof I, Simmonds P. Genotype differences in susceptibility and resistance development of hepatitis C virus to protease inhibitors telaprevir (VX-950) and danoprevir (ITMN-191). Hepatology 2011;53:1090–9.

34. GenoSure. Available at: http://www.monogrambio.com/.

35. Ge D, Fellay J, Thompson AJ, et al. Genetic variation in IL28B predicts hepatitis C treatment-induced viral clearance. Nature 2009;461:399–401.

36. Thompson AJ. Genetic factors and hepatitis C virus infection. Gastroenterology 2012;142:1335–9.

37. Thomas DL, Thio CL, Martin MP, et al. Genetic variation in IL28B and spontaneous clearance of hepatitis C virus. Nature 2009;461:798–801.

38. Neukam K, Camacho A, Caruz A, et al. Prediction of response to pegylated interferon plus ribavirin in HIV/hepatitis C virus (HCV)-coinfected patients using HCV genotype, IL28B variations, and HCV-RNA load. J Hepatol 2012;56:788–94.

39. Cisneros E, Banos I, Citores MJ, et al. Increased risk of severe hepatitis C virus recurrence after liver transplantation in patients with a T allele of IL28B rs12979860. Transplantation 2012;94:275–80.

40. Duarte-Rojo A, Veldt BJ, Goldstein DD, et al. The course of post-transplant hepatitis C infection: comparative impact of donor and recipient source of the favorable IL28B genotype and other variables. Transplantation 2012;94:197–203.
41. Eurich D, Boas-Knoop S, Bahra M, et al. Role of IL28B polymorphism in the development of hepatitis C virus-induced hepatocellular carcinoma, graft fibrosis, and post-transplant antiviral therapy. Transplantation 2012;93:644–9.
42. Fukuhara T, Taketomi A, Motomura T, et al. Variants in IL28B in liver recipients and donors correlate with response to peg-interferon and ribavirin therapy for recurrent hepatitis C. Gastroenterology 2010;139:1577–85.
43. Kawaoka T, Takahashi S, Takaki S, et al. IL28B SNP of donors and recipients can predict virological response to PEGIFN/RBV therapy in patients with recurrent hepatitis C after living donor liver transplantation. J Gastroenterol Hepatol 2012;27(9):1467–72.
44. Lange CM, Moradpour D, Doehring A, et al. Impact of donor and recipient IL28B rs12979860 genotypes on hepatitis C virus liver graft reinfection. J Hepatol 2011; 55:322–7.
45. Motomura T, Taketomi A, Fukuhara T, et al. The impact of IL28B genetic variants on recurrent hepatitis C in liver transplantation: significant lessons from a dual graft case. Am J Transplant 2011;11:1325–9.
46. Zeuzem S, Andreone P, Pol S, et al. Realize trial final results: telaprevir-based regimen for genotype 1 hepatitis C virus infection in patients with prior null response, partial response or relapse to peginterferon/ribavirin. J Hepatol 2011; 54:S3 Ref type: abstract.

Telaprevir for Chronic Hepatitis C Virus Infection

Arun B. Jesudian, MD*, Ira M. Jacobson, MD

KEYWORDS

- Hepatitis C virus • Telaprevir • Direct-acting antivirals

KEY POINTS

- Telaprevir is a recently approved direct-acting antiviral against hepatitis C virus (HCV) that works through inhibition of the NS3/4A serine protease inhibitor.
- Phase 2b and 3 studies have shown marked increase in sustained virologic response rates in both treatment-naïve and treatment-experienced patients with HCV genotype 1 treated with a telaprevir-containing regimen compared with pegylated interferon (Peg-IFN) and ribavirin alone.
- The most commonly observed side effects of telaprevir therapy are anemia to a greater degree than that observed with Peg-IFN/ribavirin alone; eczematous rash, which can be severe in a minority of patients; and anorectal discomfort.

INTRODUCTION

Approximately 3 to 4 million persons in the United States and 170 million worldwide are infected with the hepatitis C virus (HCV),[1] and up to 75% of new infections progress to chronic infection, which is a major cause of chronic liver disease.[2,3] HCV is the leading cause of death from liver disease and the most frequent indication for liver transplant in the United States.[4]

For a decade, standard of care therapy for chronic HCV genotype 1 consisted of pegylated interferon (Peg-IFN) alfa-2a or Peg-IFN alfa-2b combined with ribavirin for 48 weeks in patients with HCV genotype 1 or 24 weeks in those with HCV genotype 2 or 3.[5] Despite the improvement in efficacy over previous regimens when this therapy was introduced, the overall sustained virologic response (SVR) rate in patients with HCV genotype 1 was still only 40% to 50%.[6]

TELAPREVIR: MECHANISM OF ACTION

Determination of the structure of HCV proteins, the development of a subgenomic replicon system, and a cell culture model that enables productive HCV infection have facilitated the development of direct-acting antiviral agents.[7,8] These agents

---

Division of Gastroenterology and Hepatology, New York-Presbyterian Hospital/Weill Cornell Medical College, New York, New York, USA
* Corresponding author.
E-mail address: arun.jesudian@gmail.com

Clin Liver Dis 17 (2013) 47–62
http://dx.doi.org/10.1016/j.cld.2012.09.010
1089-3261/13/$ – see front matter © 2013 Elsevier Inc. All rights reserved.

have the potential to substantially increase rates of SVR and truncate the duration of therapy.[9]

Each step of the HCV lifecycle (**Fig. 1**) offers a potential target for direct-acting antiviral therapy. Polyprotein processing is one such step. Two viral peptidases are involved in the posttranslational processing of HCV proteins: NS2 and NS3/4A. NS3 is a multifunctional viral protein containing a serine proteinase domain in its *N*-terminal third ($\approx$180 amino acids) and a helicase/nucleoside triphosphatase domain in its *C*-terminal two-thirds. NS3 has a typical chymotrypsin-like fold, and NS4A is a cofactor of its proteinase activity. The NS3/4A serine protease catalyzes HCV polyprotein cleavage. NS3 must assemble with its cofactor NS4A to catalyze *cis*-cleavage at the NS3/4A junction and *trans*-cleavage at all downstream junctions, including NS4A–NS4B, NS4B–NS5A, and NS5A–NS5B. The cleavage sites recognized by NS3/4A protease have in common the following sequence: Asp/Glu/XXXXCys/Thr-Ser/Ala, with *trans*-cleavage occurring downstream of a cysteine residue and the *cis*-cleavage occurring downstream of a threonine residue.[9] Telaprevir is an NS3/4A serine protease inhibitor produced by Vertex Pharmaceuticals (Cambridge,

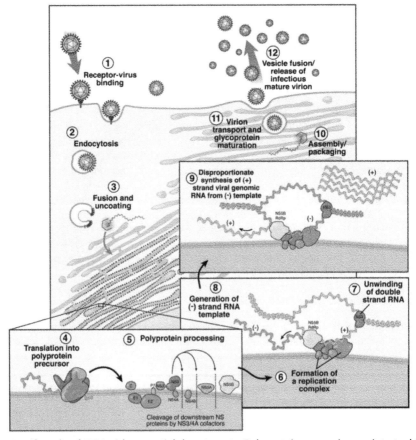

Fig. 1. Life cycle of HCV with potential drug targets. Polyprotein processing- point at which telaprevir acts. (*From* Pawlotsky JM. The hepatitis C viral life cycle as a target for new antiviral therapies. Gastroenterology 2007;132:1979–98; with permission.)

Massachusetts). It is a potent covalent orally bioavailable peptidomimetic inhibitor of NS3/4A with an α-ketoamide moiety that anchors at the enzyme active site.

PHASE 1 STUDIES

The phase 1 clinical trials for telaprevir were initially conducted in 2 parts at 2 collaborative sites in The Netherlands and 1 in Germany in 2004 to 2005.[10,11] In the first part of the initial trial, 24 healthy subjects received doses of 450 mg q8h, 750 mg q8h, and 1250 mg q12h of telaprevir for 5 days. Telaprevir was well tolerated, and no serious adverse events were reported. The second part of the trial was conducted to evaluate the safety and tolerability of ascending multiple doses of telaprevir in patients with chronic hepatitis C, and to investigate its pharmacokinetics and antiviral activity. Median HCV RNA levels in the telaprevir dose groups substantially and rapidly decreased. The median maximum change was -3.46 $\log_{10}$ IU/mL in the 450-mg q8h group, -4.77 $\log_{10}$ IU/mL in the 750-mg q8h group, and -3.49 $\log_{10}$ IU/mL in the group that received 1250 mg of telaprevir every 12 hours (q12h). All subjects in the telaprevir groups had at least a 2-$\log_{10}$ decrease in HCV RNA levels from baseline. All subjects in the 750-mg q8h group had at least a 3-$\log_{10}$ decrease. All 3 telaprevir dose groups showed similar declines in median HCV RNA levels up to day 3 of dosing. A further decrease was not evident in the 450-mg q8h and 1250-mg q12h groups, and median HCV RNA levels in those 2 dose groups increased at the end of the dosing period.

The initial rapid decline in HCV RNA was related to maximal exposure to telaprevir, and the second phase of the viral decline was sustained by trough concentrations (C_{trough}) of telaprevir. Subjects who received the 750-mg q8h regimen had an average C_{trough} of 1054 ng/mL and a 4-$\log_{10}$ or greater decrease in HCV RNA, whereas subjects who received the 450-mg q8h regimen had an average C_{trough} of 781 ng/mL with a 3-$\log_{10}$ or greater decrease in HCV RNA, and subjects who received the 1250-mg q12h regimen had an average C_{trough} of 676 ng/mL with a 3-$\log_{10}$ or greater decrease in HCV RNA.[12]

Based on these data, telaprevir at a dose of 750 mg q8h emerged as the lead dosing regimen for further trials. The virologic breakthroughs that occurred during the dosing period were related to selection of viral variants with decreased sensitivity to telaprevir and confirmed that telaprevir would need to be used in combination therapy.[12]

The resistant variants were well characterized in subsequent studies, which differentiated high-level from low-level resistant variants and defined a generally inverse relationship between degree of resistance conferred by a mutation and the replicative fitness of the resulting viral variant.[13]

Further study was undertaken to evaluate telaprevir monotherapy versus combination therapy with telaprevir and Peg-IFN. Twenty treatment-naïve patients with HCV genotype 1 were randomized to 1 of 3 treatment regimens: placebo q8h orally for 14 days and Peg-IFN weekly for 2 weeks (n = 4); telaprevir q8h orally for 14 days (n = 8); or telaprevir q8h orally for 14 days and Peg-IFN weekly for 2 weeks (n = 8). Telaprevir was dosed at 1250 mg once and then subsequent doses were 750 mg q8h. Telaprevir/Peg-IFN combination therapy resulted in a more significant viral decline during the study period, with a median change in HCV RNA from baseline to day 15 of -5.49-$\log_{10}$ compared with -3.99-$\log_{10}$ for telaprevir monotherapy and -1.09-$\log_{10}$ for Peg-IFN monotherapy.[13,14] Analysis of viral kinetics during the study period revealed a biphasic viral decline. The rapid first phase was similar in the Peg-IFN/telaprevir and telaprevir groups. The second phase of decline was more sustained in the Peg-IFN/telaprevir combination group. In the telaprevir monotherapy group, 4 patients had continued decline and 4 had viral decline followed by rebound.[14]

In the 4 patients who had viral rebound on telaprevir alone, R155K/T- and A156V/T-resistant variants were detected by sequence analysis during the initial steep decline but were replaced by V36(M/A)/R155(K/T) double-mutant variants during the rebound phase. This V36(M/A)/R155(K/T) double-mutant variant had been shown in in vitro analysis to confer higher levels of resistance and higher relative fitness.[13] All patients enrolled in the trial were offered continued therapy off-study with Peg-IFN and ribavirin after the study period, of which 19 accepted. All 8 patients initially treated in the combination Peg-IFN/telaprevir group had undetectable HCV RNA at week 12 while receiving standard of care with Peg-IFN/ribavirin compared with 5 of 8 patients who were initially treated with telaprevir monotherapy. At week 24 on standard therapy, all patients who had initially received Peg-IFN/telaprevir or telaprevir alone had achieved undetectable HCV RNA, thereby illustrating that telaprevir-resistant variants are sensitive to Peg-IFN and ribavirin.[13,14]

In logical progression, further phase 1 study was then conducted using telaprevir in combination with the current standard-of-care therapy of Peg-IFN/ribavirin. Twelve treatment-naïve subjects with chronic HCV genotype 1 were treated with telaprevir 750 mg q8h, Peg-IFN 180 µg/wk, and ribavirin 1000 or 1200 mg/d for 28 days, and then could continue treatment with Peg-IFN and ribavirin for up to 44 weeks. All 12 subjects had a decrease from baseline of at least $4\text{-}log_{10}$ and 10 subjects had a decrease greater than $5\text{-}log_{10}$. No viral breakthrough occurred. Viral sequencing analysis showed no evidence of previously identified telaprevir-resistant mutations in 10 subjects during study drug dosing. Although resistant mutations were noted in 2 subjects, their viral load continued to decline, again indicating sensitivity to Peg-IFN/ribavirin. Two subjects had undetectable HCV RNA within 8 days, and all were undetectable at 28 days. Twelve subjects continued therapy: 8 achieved an SVR, 2 had viral breakthrough, and 2 were lost to follow-up. All subjects had at least 1 adverse event, with the most frequent being influenza-like illness, fatigue, headache, nausea, anemia, depression, and pruritis.[15]

Based on this background, the PROVE (PROtease inhibition for Viral Evaluation) phase 2 trials were initiated.

PHASE 2 STUDIES
PROVE 1

PROVE 1 studied the safety and efficacy of telaprevir in combination with Peg-IFN and ribavirin (PR) in noncirrhotic treatment-naïve subjects with HCV genotype 1 in the United States (**Fig. 2**).[16] It was designed as a randomized, double-blind, placebo-controlled, multicenter (N = 37) phase 2b study. The study population included treatment-naïve subjects with chronic HCV genotype 1 aged 18 to 65 years in the United States. Exclusion criteria included infection with hepatitis B virus (HBV) or HIV, cirrhosis on biopsy within 2 years, decompensated liver disease, hepatocellular carcinoma (HCC), another cause of clinically significant liver disease, absolute neutrophil count less than $1500/mm^3$, and platelets less than $90,000/mm^3$. Most study subjects were middle-aged (mean age, 48 years) white (77%) men (63%), and 87% had a viral load greater than 800,000 IU/mL. Subjects were stratified by weight (> or ≤75 kg) and race (black or other). The study design included 4 treatment groups: (1) T12PR12 (telaprevir, 1250 mg on day 1 and then 750 mg q8h thereafter for 12 weeks with Peg-IFN, 180 µg/wk, and ribavirin, 1000 to 1200 mg/d, for the same 12 weeks; n = 17); (2) T12PR24 (telaprevir, 1250 mg on day 1 and then 750 mg q8h thereafter for 12 weeks with Peg-IFN and ribavirin, and then an additional 12 weeks Peg-IFN and ribavirin; n = 79); (3) T12PR48 (telaprevir, 1250 mg on day 1 and then 750 mg

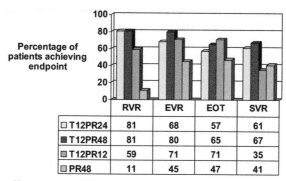

	RVR	EVR	EOT	SVR
☐ T12PR24	81	68	57	61
■ T12PR48	81	80	65	67
☐ T12PR12	59	71	71	35
☐ PR48	11	45	47	41

Fig. 2. PROVE 1 efficacy data. EOT, end of treatment; EVR, early virologic response; RVR, rapid virologic response; SVR, sustained virologic response. (*Data from* McHutchinson JG, Everson GT, Gordon SC, et al. Telaprevir with peginterferon and ribavirin for chronic HCV genotype 1 infection. N Engl J Med 2009;360(18):1827–38.)

q8h thereafter for 12 weeks with Peg-IFN and ribavirin, and then an additional 36 weeks of Peg-IFN and ribavirin; n = 79); and (4) PR48 (control group, standard of care; n = 75). Standard stopping rules applied in the PR48 control group (2-$\log_{10}$ decline in HCV RNA by week 12 of treatment and undetectable viral load at week 24). Subjects in the T12PR24 and T12PR12 groups were required to have a rapid virologic response (RVR; HCV RNA undetectable) to stop therapy at 24 or 12 weeks, respectively. If they did not achieve RVR, they were treated to 48 weeks. If breakthrough occurred (>100 IU/mL after being undetectable or increase in RNA of 1-$\log_{10}$ unit) during the first 12 weeks, then telaprevir or placebo was discontinued and the standard of care was continued. If breakthrough did occur and the viral load was greater than 1000 IU/mL, then sequencing of the NS3/4A region was performed.

SVR rates were 41% for the standard-of-care regimen (PR48), 35% in T12PR12, 61% for T12PR24, and 67% for T12PR48. Rates of RVR were also better in telaprevir-treated subjects (59%, 81%, and 81% for T12PR12, T12PR24, and T12PR48, respectively, vs 8% for PR48). Relapse was less common in subjects who received telaprevir and were treated for at least 24 weeks (2% and 6% for T12PR24 and T12PR48, respectively, vs 33% and 23% for T12PR12 and PR48, respectively). The rate of virologic breakthrough in telaprevir-treated patients was 7%, with most of the breakthroughs occurring in patients who had never cleared HCV RNA completely. In patients experiencing break-through, resistant variants were detected, with mutations including V36M, R155K (genotype 1a), or A156T (genotype 1b). V36M and R155K/T variants are observed in patients with genotype 1a because of a lower genetic barrier, because these mutations require only 1 nucleotide change in the triplet codon at the 36 and 155 positions compared with 2 changes required in genotype 1b.[13] The V36M and R155K/T variants are more fit than the A156T variant noted in patients with genotype 1b.[13]

A higher rate of discontinuation of the overall treatment regimen because of adverse events (21%) was seen in the telaprevir-based groups (11%) versus control patients, with an increased frequency of rash, pruritus, nausea, diarrhea, and anemia noted. Twelve patients (7%) who received telaprevir developed severe rash and discontinued therapy compared with 1 control patient (1%). Erythropoiesis-stimulating agents were prohibited for the first 12 weeks of treatment. The mean decline in hemoglobin was 3 g/dL in the control group, with an incremental rate of hemoglobin decline of 0.5 to 1 g/dL more in telaprevir-treated patients. After telaprevir was discontinued the hemoglobin increased.

PROVE 1 demonstrated superiority of combination therapy over standard of care and illustrated that with combination therapy a shorter treatment course could be considered. It raised RVR as a required criterion for stopping therapy at earlier time points than the standard 48 weeks. Rash and anemia emerged as the most common side effects of therapy.[16]

PROVE 2

PROVE 2 was the European counterpart to PROVE 1. It evaluated the safety and efficacy of telaprevir in combination with Peg-IFN with or without ribavirin in noncirrhotic treatment-naïve patients with HCV genotype 1.[17] It was designed as a multicenter, randomized, partially double-blind, placebo-controlled phase 2b trial.

The patients were divided into 4 treatment groups (N = 334): T12PR12, T12PR24, T12P12 (telaprevir and Peg-IFN only), and standard-of-care regimen PR48. The ribavirin-free arm (T12P12) was distinct from PROVE 1, as was all 4 treatment arms having an equivalent number of patients. An RVR was not required for patients to stop therapy at the predefined stopping point defined in each treatment arm. Instead, patients in the T12PR24, T12PR12, and T12P12 groups were required to have undetectable HCV RNA levels at the last study visit before the planned end of treatment, which was week 10 for the T12PR12 and T12P12 groups and week 20 for the T12PR24 group, or they continued Peg-IFN/ribavirin for 48 weeks. SVR rates were 46% in the control group (PR), 36% in the T12P12 group, 60% in T12PR12 group, and 69% in T12PR24 group. RVR rates were 13% for PR48, 50% for T12P12, 69% for T12PR24, and 80% for T12PR12. Relapse occurred in 22% of controls, 48% of patients treated without ribavirin (T12P12), 14% of the T12PR24 group, and 30% of the T12PR12 group. A multivariate analysis showed that treatment group and baseline HCV RNA were the only 2 variables significantly associated with SVR.

HCV virus with low-level resistance was found at baseline in 1% of subjects. Among subjects with viral breakthrough who had sequencing performed, wild-type virus was noted in 5%, low-level resistance in 41%, and high-level resistance in 55%. Among subjects who experienced relapse who had sequencing performed, wild-type virus was noted in 5%, low-level resistance in 79%, and high-level resistance in 17%.

The median time to appearance of rash of any severity in the telaprevir-based groups was 9 to 12 days. Severe (grade 3) rash was found in 7% of patients (6 of 81) in the T12PR24 group, 6% (5 of 82) in the T12PR12 group, and 3% (2 of 78) in the T12P12 group, but was not seen in the PR48 group. Twelve of the 163 patients (7%) in the combined T12PR24 and T12PR12 groups discontinued treatment because of rash.

PROVE 2 confirmed that telaprevir is effective and has an acceptable tolerability profile in combination therapy for the treatment of treatment-naïve subjects with HCV genotype 1 and that the clinical viral breakthrough that occurred during the dosing period was related to selection of viral variants with decreased sensitivity to telaprevir. It highlighted the importance of ribavirin in the treatment regimen. It revealed that baseline viral load was predictive of response even with telaprevir therapy.[17]

PROVE 3

PROVE 3 was undertaken to evaluate telaprevir's efficacy (**Fig. 3**) in patients with HCV infection who had not had a sustained response to an initial full course of treatment with Peg-IFN and ribavirin (ie, prior treatment failures).[18] It was an international, randomized, partially placebo-controlled, partially double-blind phase 2 study. The study population included subjects with HCV genotype 1 aged 18 to 70 years who had been previously treated with Peg-IFN/ribavirin for at least 12 weeks and did not have a SVR (**Fig. 4**). They were stratified by type of treatment failure: nonresponse,

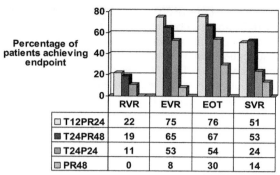

Fig. 3. PROVE 3 efficacy data. (*Data from* McHutchinson JG, Manns MP, Muir AJ, et al. Telaprevir for previously treated chronic HCV infection. N Engl J Med 2010;362(14):1292–303.)

relapse, and breakthrough; 57% were considered to previously have had nonresponse, 36% relapse, and 7% breakthrough. Exclusion criteria included chronic HBV, HIV, cirrhosis on biopsy within 2 years, decompensated liver disease, HCC, another cause of clinically significant liver disease, absolute neutrophil count less than 1500/mm^3, and platelet count less than 100,000/mm^3. Subjects were required to have had a liver biopsy within 3 years. Unlike PROVE 1 and 2, PROVE 3 included patients with cirrhosis, which constituted 16% of the study population. Patients were assigned to 4 treatment groups: T12PR24, T24PR48, T24PR24, and PR48. Those in the control group (PR48) were allowed to roll over and receive telaprevir after study conclusion. Telaprevir was dosed at 1125 mg on day 1 and then 750 mg orally q8h. Stopping rules included breakthrough between weeks 4 and 24; less than a 1-log$_{10}$ drop by week 4 in the control group; HCV greater than 30 IU/mL at week 4 in the telaprevir-treated subjects; less than a 2-log$_{10}$ decline at week 12; and detectable virus at week 24.

The T12PR24 and T24PR48 regimens were most efficacious and not statistically different from one another, with SVR rates of 51% and 53% respectively, versus 24% with T24P24 and 14% with PR48. However, discontinuation of therapy because of adverse events was less common in the T12PR24 group than in the T24PR48 group. Rates of SVR were higher among subjects who had a previous relapse (T12PR24, 69%; T24PR48, 76%; T24P24, 42%; and PR48, 20%) than among those who experienced no response to previous treatment (T12PR24, 39%; T24PR48, 38%; T24P24, 11%; PR48, 9%). Less relapse was seen among the subjects in the T12PR24 and

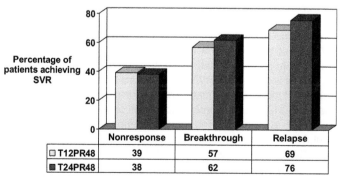

Fig. 4. PROVE 3 SVR by prior treatment response. (*Data from* McHutchinson JG, Manns MP, Muir AJ, et al. Telaprevir for previously treated chronic HCV infection. N Engl J Med 2010;362(14):1292–303.)

T24PR48 arms, with relapse rates of 30% and 13%, respectively, versus 53% in both the T24P24 and PR48 groups. For subjects in the T24PR48 group who actually completed treatment, relapse rates were 4% overall, 4% for patients with no previous response, and 0% for patients with a previous relapse. More breakthroughs were seen in patients with genotype 1a than 1b, with rates of 24% versus 11%. In a subanalysis, patients with and without cirrhosis had equivalent rates of SVR in this study.

Logistic regression analysis showed that a SVR was significantly associated with assignment to the T12PR24 or T24PR48 group, an undetectable HCV RNA level during a previous period of treatment with Peg-IFN alfa and ribavirin, and low baseline viral load (<800,000 IU/mL). Most subjects who discontinued therapy because of a stopping rule had the V36M/R155K double variant; all but one of the subjects had infection with HCV genotype 1a.

Again, relapse occurred less frequently with the T24PR48 regimen than with the T12PR24 regimen, and rates of SVR were similar in the T12PR24 and T24PR48 groups. However, discontinuation of therapy because of adverse events was less common in the T12PR24 group than in the T24PR48 group. The overall efficacy and safety results indicate that the T12PR24 regimen provided a better risk/benefit profile than the T24PR48 regimen.[18] This finding raised the question of whether selected patients who are tolerating treatment and have a significant risk of relapse (eg, those with genotype 1a) might optimize their treatment with a total of 48 weeks of therapy, perhaps with an initial 12 weeks of telaprevir. This hypothesis is, in fact, what was studied in phase 3.

PHASE 3 STUDIES
A New Direction in HCV Care: A Study of Treatment-Naïve Hepatitis C Patients with Telaprevir (ADVANCE)

ADVANCE was the larger of 2 phase 3 trials of telaprevir in treatment-naïve patients with HCV genotype 1.[19] In addition to establishing the safety and efficacy of telaprevir for purposes of registration, it had 2 important goals: first, to explore an 8-week rather than a 12-week course of telaprevir to assess whether the incidence or severity of side effects, particularly rash, could be reduced while preserving efficacy; second, to assess the capacity to truncate therapy to 24 weeks in patients with robust viral responses and still attain high rates of SVR with minimal relapse.

ADVANCE was a 3-arm, double-blind, randomized study that was placebo-controlled for telaprevir. The study population (N = 1088) consisted of treatment-naïve subjects with HCV genotype 1 and included subjects with advanced fibrosis (21%) (ie, bridging fibrosis or compensated cirrhosis). Patients in the telaprevir arms received either 12 or 8 weeks of telaprevir at a dose of 750 mg q8h, Peg-IFN, and ribavirin, followed by Peg-IFN and ribavirin alone (T8PR or T12PR). Patients who attained undetectable HCV RNA at both weeks 4 and 12 were defined as having had extended RVR (eRVR), and were assigned to stop after total treatment of 24 weeks. In contrast, patients who did not experience eRVR were treated for up to 48 weeks.

Stopping rules included discontinuation of telaprevir alone after 4 weeks if HCV RNA was more than 1000 IU/mL, discontinuation of all treatment for less than a 2-$\log_{10}$ decline in HCV RNA at week 12, and discontinuation of all therapy for detectability of HCV RNA at 24 weeks or any time thereafter.

SVR rates of 75% and 69% for T12PR and T8PR, respectively (**Fig. 5**), compared with 44% in controls confirmed the superiority of telaprevir combination therapy over the current standard of care (P<.001 for T12PR or T8PR vs PR). Relapse rates were 9% in each of the telaprevir groups and 28% in the control patients. Patients in the T12PR and T8PR groups had RVR rates of 68% and 67%, respectively, and

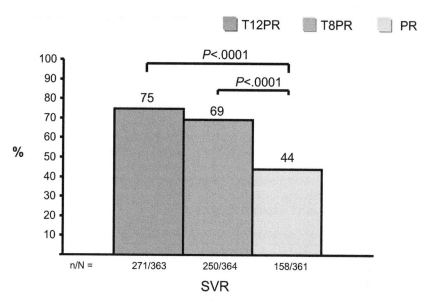

Fig. 5. ADVANCE SVR rates. (*Data from* Jacobson IM, McHutchison JG, Dusheiko G, et al. Telaprevir for previously untreated chronic hepatitis C virus infection. N Engl J Med 2011;364(25):2405–16.)

eRVR rates of 58% and 57%, versus only 9% and 8% of controls. The patients with eRVR were those assigned to 24 weeks of treatment; these patients had SVR rates of 89% (T12PR) and 83% (T8PR). Of the small number of patients who received PR for 48 weeks after attaining eRVR, 97% had SVR. Patients who failed eRVR had SVR rates of 54%, 50%, and 39% in the T12PR, T8PR, and PR groups. Subset analyses showed that African Americans who received PR had SVR of 25% versus 62% with T12PR, and patients with advanced fibrosis had an increase in SVR from 33% to 62%.

The rate of virologic failure, defined by the meeting of one of the stopping rules or having an HCV RNA level greater than 1000 IU/mL at week 12 even if HCV RNA declined by 2 logs during the first 12 weeks, was 3% in both the T12 and T8 groups and was associated with the emergence of variants with a high level of resistance to telaprevir. After week 12, during Peg-IFN/ribavirin, treatment failure was somewhat higher in T8PR (10%) compared with T12PR (5%), and associated with wild-type and lower-level telaprevir-resistant variants. The rate of virologic failure with PR was 32%. These observations suggest that the main benefit of T12 compared with T8, reflected in the slightly higher rate of SVR of T12 (the study was not powered to demonstrate a statistical difference between T12 and T8), was more efficient clearance of wild-type and low-level resistant variants with the additional 4 weeks of telaprevir.[20]

Overall rates of treatment discontinuation for adverse events occurred in 10%, 10%, and 7% of patients in T12PR, T8PR, and PR, respectively. During the first 12 weeks of therapy, telaprevir/placebo alone was stopped in 11%, 7%, and 1%, respectively, because of adverse events overall. Telaprevir was associated with an increase in rash and anemia, and with diarrhea, pruritus, and nausea. Grade 3 rash occurred in 6%, 3%, and 1% of patients, respectively. The rash was primarily eczematous clinically and histologically. Severe rash was managed by sequentially discontinuing telaprevir, followed by ribavirin 7 days later if considered necessary, and then Peg-IFN for continued progression. Severe rash events led to discontinuation of telaprevir/placebo in 7%, 5%, and 1%, respectively. In contrast, discontinuation of all study drugs for rash events seldom occurred (1.4%, 0.5%, and 0%, respectively). The rash resolved on discontinuation.[19] The rash management plan was credited with a lower rate of overall treatment discontinuation for rash than occurred in the phase 2 program.

A nadir hemoglobin of less than 10 g/dL occurred in 38% of patients treated with telaprevir and 14% of controls, whereas nadir hemoglobin less than 8.5 g/dL occurred in 9% of patients treated with telaprevir and 2% of controls. As per the protocol, anemia was managed with ribavirin dose modifications, and erythropoiesis-stimulating agents were not allowed. Discontinuation of all drugs because of anemia events occurred in 1%, 3%, and 1% of patients in T12PR, T8PR, and PR, respectively, and 4%, 2%, and 0% of patients, respectively, discontinued telaprevir/placebo only. By 24 weeks of therapy, hemoglobin levels were comparable among patients who had initially received telaprevir and controls. Re-treatment with only 8 weeks of telaprevir was not associated with less discontinuation of the entire treatment regimen from adverse events than was 12 weeks (8% vs 7%).[19]

Illustrating the Effects of Combination Therapy with Telaprevir (ILLUMINATE)

The ADVANCE study strongly suggested that 24 weeks of total therapy was sufficient in patients with eRVR, an inference derived from the high rates of SVR and low rates of relapse in patients with eRVR treated for 24 weeks. To support this concept, the ILLUMINATE trial was undertaken.[21] It was an open-label multicenter (N = 74) phase 3 study. Treatment-naïve subjects with HCV genotype 1 treated with 12 weeks of triple therapy (telaprevir, Peg-IFN, and ribavirin) and those who achieved an eRVR were randomized at week 20 to receive either 24 or 48 weeks of total Peg-IFN/ribavirin therapy to show noninferiority of the 24-week treatment course. Patients who did not achieve an eRVR continued 48 weeks of therapy. The study population included patients with cirrhosis (11%).

Noninferiority of the 24-week treatment regimen among subjects who achieved eRVR was established by SVR rates of 92% for 24 weeks versus 88% for 48 weeks of therapy. Overall SVR in the intention-to-treat analysis was 72%. Permanent discontinuation of therapy because of adverse events occurred in 17.4% of subjects and was more common in the 48-week treatment group. ILLUMINATE affirmed the foundation for response-guided therapy in telaprevir-containing combination treatment of HCV.[21]

REALIZE

The REALIZE trial (Re-treatment of Patients with Telaprevir-based Regimen to Optimize Outcomes) was conducted to further define telaprevir-based therapy in subjects for whom a previous course of Peg-IFN and ribavirin failed.[22] Subjects were assigned to 3 treatment arms: (1) telaprevir dosed at 750 mg q8h for 12 weeks in combination with standard doses of Peg-IFN and ribavirin, followed by 36 weeks of treatment with Peg-IFN and ribavirin alone; (2) a delayed start arm, composed of 4 weeks of treatment with Peg-IFN and ribavirin, followed by telaprevir dosed at 750 mg q8h for 12 weeks in combination with standard doses of Peg-IFN and ribavirin, followed by another 32 weeks of Peg-IFN and ribavirin alone; and (3) a control arm with standard doses of Peg-IFN and ribavirin dosed for 48 weeks.

Overall, SVR occurred in 65% of telaprevir recipients and 17% of controls. No significant difference in SVR rates were seen between patients in the delayed start arm and those who started all 3 drugs simultaneously. As expected, a gradient of SVR occurred, so that patients with the highest degree of intrinsic responsiveness to interferon (ie, relapsers) had the highest rate of SVR (86%). Partial responders, those with a greater than 2-log_{10} reduction in HCV RNA at week 12 previously, had an SVR in 57%, and null responders, who had a less than 2-log_{10} decline in HCV RNA at week 12 previously, had an SVR in 31% (**Fig. 6**).

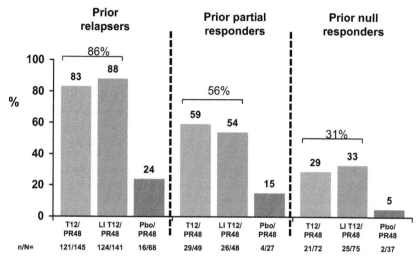

Fig. 6. REALIZE SVR rates. (*Data from* Zeuzem S, Andreone P, Pol S, et al. Telaprevir for retreatment of HCV infection. N Engl J Med 2011;364(25):2417–28.)

An important subanalysis of this trial showed that, among relapsers, cirrhosis did not adversely affect SVR rates. However, in prior partial responders with cirrhosis, the SVR rate was reduced to 34% and, even more impactfully, prior null responders with cirrhosis had an SVR rate of only 14%.

Analysis of the lead-in arm of the REALIZE trial evaluated the association between degree of HCV RNA decline after the 4-week lead-in period of Peg-IFN/ribavirin and the subsequent likelihood of SVR.[23] In relapsers, SVR rates were 62% in those who had less than a 1-log_{10} decline in HCV RNA at week 4 compared with 94% in those with a decline of 1-log_{10} or greater. In partial responders, SVR rates were 56% and 50%, respectively. The greatest impact was observed in prior null responders, with SVR rates of 15% and 54%, respectively.

EXTEND

The capacity of HCV to become resistant to direct-acting antiviral agents in general, including protease inhibitors, manifests itself in the resistant variants that are usually detectable in patients with virologic failure or breakthrough on therapy with telaprevir. Considerable concern exists about the long-term fate and clinical impact of these resistant variants. If these variants are persistent, they could theoretically have an adverse impact on treatment outcomes if patients for whom a prior course of therapy with a protease inhibitor failed are being considered for retreatment with future regimens containing the same or similar drugs. The EXTEND trial was conducted as a 3-year virology follow-up study on subjects from the phase 2 and 3 telaprevir trials. An interim analysis of patients in the phase 2 studies, who hence had a longer follow-up period as of late 2010, showed a durable SVR (99%) with telaprevir-based therapy and a reversion to wild-type virus in subjects who had developed telaprevir resistance on therapy. Evaluation of subjects who had viral variants (amino acid positions 36, 54, 155, and 156) associated with decreased telaprevir susceptibility at treatment failure showed that at a median of 25 months after treatment, the resistant variants had cleared in 89% of subjects as determined by population sequencing, which requires that at least 20% of the viral population consist of a given variant.[24] These results were verified in a subset of patients evaluated using more sensitive clonal sequencing. This analysis is planned to continue, and long-term monitoring studies such as these should be considered important components of trials evaluating new direct-acting antiviral agents.

FURTHER STUDIES
Retreatment

Building on the results of the studies using telaprevir-based therapy in treatment-experienced patients, investigators in the PROVE studies selected 117 patients in the placebo arms who either did not experience response or experienced relapse with Peg-IFN/ribavirin, and rolled them over into treatment with telaprevir-containing regimens.[25] The initial protocol was 12 weeks of telaprevir/Peg-IFN/ribavirin followed by an additional 12 weeks of Peg-IFN/ribavirin. The protocol was changed during the study so that prior null responders had Peg-IFN extended to week 48, whereas all other patients received either 24 total weeks of therapy if HCV RNA was undetectable at weeks 4 and 12 or 48 weeks of therapy if HCV RNA was detectable at weeks 4 or 12. The overall SVR rate was 59%. SVR was achieved in 37% (19/51) of prior null responders, 55% (16/29) of prior partial responders, 75% (6/8) in prior breakthroughs, and 97% (28/29) of prior relapsers.

The observations in relapsers helped establish the recommendation on the product label to truncate total therapy to 24 weeks in the event of an eRVR, even though only 48 weeks of therapy was evaluated in the phase 3 REALIZE study.

Effect of ribavirin dose reduction

Retrospective analysis was performed on the treatment-naïve patients in the ADVANCE and ILLUMINATE trials and the treatment-experienced patients in the REALIZE trial who received the telaprevir-containing regimen to assess the effect of ribavirin dose-reduction on SVR rates.[26] Of the treatment-naïve patients, 50% required a ribavirin dose reduction, including 45% with a reduction to 600 mg/d or lower. In these patients, 75% of those reduced to 800 to 1000 mg of ribavirin and 74% of those reduced to 600 mg/d or less experienced an SVR, compared with 79% who did not require a ribavirin dose reduction. In the treatment-experienced patients, ribavirin dose reduction was required in 39% of the prior relapsers, 31% of the prior partial responders, and 18% of the prior null responders in the telaprevir arms. Of the prior relapsers, SVR was achieved in 90% who had ribavirin dose reduction to 600 mg/d or lower and in 84% who had ribavirin dose reduction to 800 to 1000 mg/d, compared with 82% in those who did not require ribavirin dose reduction. In prior partial responders, 62% of those who had a ribavirin dose reduction to 600 mg/d or lower achieved SVR compared with 50% who had a reduction to 800 to 1000 mg/d and 62% who did not require dose reduction. Finally, SVR rates in prior null responders were 22% in those who had reduction to 600 mg/d or less of ribavirin, 50% in those reduced to 800 to 1000 mg/d, and 31% who did not require dose reduction. Collectively, these observations have reassured clinicians that ribavirin dose reductions for anemia do not substantially compromise the chance of SVR.

Safety of use in cirrhosis

Given the small number of patients with cirrhosis included in the aforementioned phase 3 trials, further study investigated the safety of treating these patients with a telaprevir-containing regimen.[27] In the French Early Access Program (ANRS C020-CUPIC), 169 patients with compensated Child-Pugh class A HCV genotype 1 cirrhosis were treated with telaprevir in combination with Peg-IFN alfa-2a and ribavirin. Patients were treated for a median of 16 weeks before abstract publication. Overall, 51% of patients experienced a serious adverse event. Discontinuation of treatment medications occurred in 12% of patients. Grade 2 anemia was observed in 32% of patients, whereas grade 3 to 4 anemia was observed in 14%. With the proviso that ribavirin dose reductions were seldom implemented in these patients, more than half required erythropoietin administration for anemia and 19% required blood transfusions. Grade 3 to 4 anemia was observed in 12% of patients, whereas grade 3 to 4 thrombocytopenia was observed in 22%. Finally, 7% experienced grade 3 rash, whereas 2% died while being treated.

Dosing Frequency and Interferon Preparation Considerations

A recent study investigated the safety, tolerability, and pharmacokinetics of telaprevir dosed in the usual 750 mg q8h interval and 1125 mg q12h in combination with either Peg-IFN alfa-2a or Peg-IFN alfa-2b.[28] In this study, 161 treatment-naïve patients were randomized to receive 1 of the 2 telaprevir dosing regimens combined with either Peg-IFN alpha-2a or Peg-IFN alpha-2b and ribavirin. All patients received triple therapy for 12 weeks followed by either 12 or 36 additional weeks of Peg-IFN/ribavirin based on viral response. No significant difference was seen in SVR rates among the groups (81%–85%), leading investigators to conclude that either telaprevir dosing frequency or type of Peg-IFN alpha was acceptable. Twice-daily telaprevir dosing is being evaluated in a larger trial.

Use in HIV/HCV coinfection

Telaprevir in combination with Peg-IFN/ribavirin is also being studied in the treatment of HIV/HCV genotype 1–coinfected individuals, a patient population with historically low response rates to treatment with Peg-IFN/ribavirin alone.[29] In a phase 2 trial, 13 coinfected patients with CD4 T-cell counts greater than 500 cells/mm^3 not currently on antiretroviral therapy (ART) and 47 coinfected patients on ARTs (24 on efavirenz + tenofovir + emtricitabine and 23 on ritonavir-boosted atazanavir + either lamivudine or emtricitabine) were randomized to receive either telaprevir with Peg-IFN alpha-2a/ribavirin or placebo with Peg-IFN alpha-2a/ribavirin. Triple therapy was given for 12 weeks, with Peg-IFN/ribavirin continued through week 48. Patients taking efavirenz had their dose of telaprevir increased to 1125 mg 3 times daily to compensate for a known drug interaction that lowers the level of telaprevir. Patients on atazanavir were given the standard dose of telaprevir, 750 mg 3 times daily.

Overall, 74% of patients taking the telaprevir-containing regimen achieved sustained virologic response 12, or persistently undetectable HCV RNA at 12 weeks after the completion of therapy (SVR12), compared with 45% of those taking Peg-IFN/ribavirin alone. In the patients not taking ARTs, the SVR12 rates were 71% and 33%, respectively. In patients taking efavirenz, SVR12 was seen in 69% of those treated with telaprevir compared with 50% of those in the Peg-IFN/ribavirin–alone arm. In patients taking atazanavir, SVR12 was seen in 80% of those in the telaprevir group compared with 50% of those in the placebo group. No HIV viral rebound was observed during the study. Three patients taking telaprevir discontinued treatment because of adverse events compared with none in the Peg-IFN/ribavirin–alone groups. These early data suggest that the efficacy and safety of HIV/HCV-coinfected patients may parallel those seen in HCV-monoinfected patients.

Efficacy in HCV genotype 2 and 3

The antiviral activity or telaprevir alone or in combination with Peg-IFN/ribavirin was recently studied in HCV genotypes 2 and 3.[30] In this randomized, multicenter trial, 23 patients with HCV genotype 2 and 26 patients with HCV genotype 3 were enrolled. Levels of HCV RNA were observed to decrease in all patients with HCV genotype 2, including those who received telaprevir monotherapy. In patients with genotype 2, SVR rates were 56% in those treated with telaprevir monotherapy followed by Peg-IFN/ribavirin for 24 weeks, 89% in those treated with Peg-IFN/ribavirin alone, and 100% in those treated with the 3-drug combination. In patients with genotype 3, telaprevir monotherapy had limited activity in terms of viral response, and addition of telaprevir did not increase the SVR rates above those associated with Peg-IFN/ribavirin alone.

CURRENT PRESCRIBING GUIDELINES AND CONSIDERATIONS

The use of a protease inhibitor in conjunction with Peg-IFN and ribavirin can be considered the new standard of care in patients infected with HCV genotype 1. Telaprevir was approved by the U.S. Food and Drug Administration (FDA) in May 2011 for the treatment of chronic HCV genotype 1 infection. The medication is available in oral tablet form and is to be given at a dose of 750 mg to be taken 3 times daily every 7 to 9 hours with a meal or snack containing 20 g of fat, in combination with Peg-IFN/ribavirin therapy.[31] Patients must receive the 3-drug regimen for 12 weeks, followed by response-guided therapy of 12 or 36 additional weeks of Peg-IFN/ribavirin, depending on viral response and prior response. For treatment-naïve patients and prior relapsers, those with undetectable HCV RNA at weeks 4 and 12 (eRVR) are instructed to undergo therapy with 12 additional weeks of Peg-IFN/ribavirin. The exception to this guideline is treatment-naïve patients with cirrhosis and undetectable HCV RNA at weeks 4 and 12, in whom 36 additional weeks of Peg-IFN/ribavirin is suggested. Many clinicians, including the authors, also recommend 48 weeks of total therapy in prior relapsers even when eRVR has been attained. For prior partial and null responders, all patients should receive 12 weeks of the 3-drug regimen, followed by 36 weeks of Peg-IFN/ribavirin. Discontinuation is recommended for patients with HCV RNA greater than 1000 IU/mL at week 4 or 12, or detectable HCV RNA at week 24. Retrospective analysis of the ADVANCE, ILLUMINATE, and REALIZE trials has now clearly shown that HCV RNA level greater than 1000 IU/mL at week 4 accurately predicted treatment failure, with 24 of 25 patients already experiencing viral breakthrough,[32] and none going on to achieve SVR despite continuation of Peg-IFN/ribavirin past week 4 in these studies.

Patients should be monitored during therapy with follow-up visits and laboratory testing, including complete blood cell count, chemistry, liver function tests, and thyroid-stimulating hormone, as per current standard of care. A greater mean level of hemoglobin decline than traditionally seen with Peg-IFN and ribavirin should be anticipated.[16,19] Anemia should be managed with ribavirin dose reductions before discontinuation of therapy. Although erythropoiesis-stimulating agents were not allowed in development programs and are not FDA-approved, they can be considered in patients on an individualized basis.

An eczematous rash may occur. Severe rash, such as that involving more than 50% of the body surface area or any evidence of mucosal ulceration, should be managed with sequential discontinuation of drug therapy as necessary, with telaprevir discontinued first, followed by ribavirin 7 days later as necessary, and Peg-IFN thereafter if continued progression is seen. Therapy need not be stopped all at once unless necessary in the clinician's judgment.[19] Although 12 weeks of telaprevir therapy is preferred, it may be discontinued at week 8 without substantial impairment of potential SVR.[19]

Because telaprevir is a potent inhibitor of the cytochrome enzyme CYP3A, it is contraindicated for concurrent use with medications that are highly dependent on CYP3A for clearance. Medications of note include lovastatin, simvastatin, and atorvastatin. Similarly, concurrent use of medications that strongly induce CYP3A should be avoided because they lead to reduced efficacy. Because exposure to ethinyl estradiol may be reduced when telaprevir is coadministered, hormonal contraceptives should not used as 1 of the 2 required methods of contraception during Peg-IFN/ribavirin therapy while telaprevir is being given and for 2 weeks after telaprevir is discontinued. Clinicians should consult the list of contraindicated drugs and the more extensive list of drugs with potential interactions available in the telaprevir package insert. Dose reduction and telaprevir monotherapy are strictly prohibited to minimize the emergence of viral resistance.

The treatment of prior null responders with telaprevir deserves particular mention. The success rates reported in these patients represent a more efficacious option than any prior treatment regimen. However, the price of treatment failure with telaprevir (or any protease inhibitor) is the high likelihood that the patient will be left with resistant variants. This circumstance is particularly notable in prior null responders, in whom the SVR rates of just greater than 30% must be balanced against the high chance of leaving patients for whom such treatment fails—which is most of this subpopulation—with resistant variants. In the risk/benefit profile pertaining to these patients, those with advanced fibrosis would seem to constitute the prior null responders in whom the most compelling argument for retreatment exists. As with all patients in the new treatment era, the concept of resistance, and the basic aspects of what is understood about its potential implications, must be conveyed in a manner understandable to the patient.

REFERENCES

1. Dienstag JL, McHutchison JG. American Gastroenterological Association technical review on the management of hepatitis C. Gastroenterology 2006;130:231–64.
2. World Health Organization, Hepatitis C. World Health Organization; 2000. Available at: http://www.who.int/mediacentre/factsheets/fs165/en. Accessed September 6, 2012.
3. El-Serag HB, Mason AC. Rising incidence of hepatocellular carcinoma in the United States. N Engl J Med 1999;340:745–50.
4. Kim WR. The burden of Hepatitis C in the United States. Hepatology 2002; 36(Suppl):S30–4.
5. Ghany MG, Strader DB, Thomas DL, et al. AASLD practice guidelines: diagnosis, management, and treatment of hepatitis C: an update. Hepatology 2009;49:1335–75.
6. Jacobson IM. Treatment options for patients with chronic hepatitis C not responding to antiviral therapy. Clin Gastroenterol Hepatol 2009;7:921–30.
7. Lohmann V, Körner F, Koch J, et al. Replication of subgenomic hepatitis C virus RNAs in a hepatoma cell line. Science 1999;285:110–3.
8. Lindenbach BD, Evans MJ, Syder AJ, et al. Complete replication of hepatitis C virus in cell culture. Science 2005;309:623–6.
9. Pawlotsky JM. The hepatitis C viral life cycle as a target for new antiviral therapies. Gastroenterology 2007;132:1979–98.
10. Perni RB, Almquist SJ, Byrn RA, et al. Preclinical profile of VX-950, a potent, selective, and orally bioavailable inhibitor of hepatitis C virus NS3-4A serine protease. Antimicrob Agents Chemother 2006;50:899–909.
11. Forestier N, Reesnik HW, Weegink CJ, et al. Antiviral activity of Telaprevir (VX-950) and peginterferon alfa-2a in patients with hepatitis C. Hepatology 2007;46:640–8.
12. Reesink HW. Rapid decline of viral RNA in hepatitis C patients treated with VX-950: a phase 1b, placebo-controlled, randomized study. Gastroenterology 2006;131:997–1002.
13. Kieffer TL, Sarrazin C, Miller JS, et al. Telaprevir and pegylated interferon-alpha-2a inhibit wild-type and resistant genotype 1 hepatitis c virus replication in patients. Hepatology 2007;46:631–9.
14. Forestier N, Reesink HW, Weegink CJ, et al. Antiviral activity of telaprevir (VX-950) and peginterferon alfa-2a in patients with hepatitis C. Hepatology 2007;46:640–7.
15. Lawitz E, Rodriguez-Torres M, Muir AJ, et al. Antiviral effects and safety of telaprevir, peginterferon alfa-2a, and ribavirin for 28 days in hepatitis C patients. J Hepatol 2008;49:163–9.

16. McHutchinson JG, Everson GT, Gordon SC, et al. Telaprevir with peginterferon and ribavirin for chronic HCV genotype 1 infection. N Engl J Med 2009;360(18):1827–38.
17. Hezode C, Forestier N, Dusheiko G, et al. Telaprevir and peginterferon with or without ribavirin for chronic HCV infection. N Engl J Med 2009;360(18):1839–50.
18. McHutchinson JG, Manns MP, Muir AJ, et al. Telaprevir for previously treated chronic HCV infection. N Engl J Med 2010;362(14):1292–303.
19. Jacobson IM, McHutchison JG, Dusheiko G, et al. Telaprevir for previously untreated chronic hepatitis C virus infection. N Engl J Med 2011;364(25):2405–16.
20. Kieffer TL, Bartels G, Sullivan J, et al. Clinical virology results from telaprevir phase 3 study ADVANCE. AASLD 2010 Annual Meeting, October 30–November 3, 2010, Boston, MA.
21. Sherman KE, Flamm SL, Afdhal NH, et al. Telaprevir in combination with peginterferon alfa2a and ribavirin for 24 or 48 weeks in treatment-naïve genotype 1 HCV patients who achieved an extended rapid viral response: final results of phase 3 ILLUMINATE study. AASLD 2010 Annual Meeting, October 30–November 3, 2010, Boston, MA.
22. Zeuzem S, Andreone P, Pol S, et al. Telaprevir for retreatment of HCV infection. N Engl J Med 2011;364(25):2417–28.
23. Foster GR, Zeuzem S, Andreone P, et al. Subanalyses of the telaprevir lead-in arm in the REALIZE study: response at week 4 is not a substitute for prior null response categorization. J Hepatol 2011;54(Suppl 1):S3–4.
24. Zeuzem S, Sulkowski MS, Zoulim F, et al. Long-term follow-up of patients with chronic hepatitis C treated with telaprevir in combination with peginterferon alfa-2a and ribavirin: interim analysis of the EXTEND Study. Presented at the 61st Annual Meeting of the American Association for the Study of Liver Diseases (AASLD 2010). Boston, October 29–November 2, 2010.
25. Muir AJ, Poordad FF, McHutchison JG, et al. Retreatment with telaprevir combination therapy in hepatitis C patients with well-characterized prior treatment response. Hepatology 2011;54(5):1538–46.
26. Sulkowski MS, Roberts S, Afdhal NH, et al. Ribavirin dose modification in treatment-naïve and previously treated patients who received telaprevir combination treatment: no impact on sustained virologic response in phase 3 studies. EASL, April 18–22, 2012, Barcelona, Spain.
27. Hezode C, Dorival C, Zoulim F, et al. Safelty of telaprevir or boceprevir in combination with peginterferon alfa/ribavirin, in cirrhotic nonresponders. First results of the French early access program (ANRS CO20-CUPIC). EASL, April 18–22, 2012, Barcelona, Spain.
28. Marcellin P, Forns X, Goeser T, et al. Telaprevir is effective given every 8 or 12 hours with ribavirin and peginterferon alfa-2a or -2b to patients with chronic hepatitis C. Gastroenterology 2011;140:459–68.
29. Dieterich D, Soriano V, Sherman K, et al. Telaprevir in combination with pegylated interferon-alfa-2a + ribavirin in HCV/HIV-coinfected patients: a 24-week treatment interim analysis. Presented at the 19th Conference on Retroviruses and Opportunistic Infections (CROI 2012). Seattle, March 5–8, 2012.
30. Foster GR, Hézode C, Bronowicki JP, et al. Telaprevir alone or with peginterferon and ribavirin reduces HCV RNA in patients with chronic genotype 2 but not genotype 3 infections. Gastroenterology 2011;141:881–9.
31. Incivek [package insert]. Cambridge (MA): Vertex Pharmaceuticals; 2011.
32. Jacobson IM, Bartels DJ, Gritz L, et al. Futility rules in telaprevir combination treatment. EASL, April 18–22, 2012, Barcelona, Spain.

Boceprevir and Treatment of Chronic Hepatitis C

Paul Y. Kwo, MD

KEYWORDS

- Boceprevir • Peginterferon • Ribavirin • Hepatitis C

KEY POINTS

- The addition of boceprevir to peginterferon and ribavirin has improved sustained response rates markedly.
- Boceprevir is effective in treatment naïve, relapsers, partial responders, and null responders. Those with advanced fibrosis require 44 weeks of boceprevir therapy after a 4-week peg/ribavirin lead-in.
- The main side effect with boceprevir is anemia, and ribavirin dose reduction is an effective strategy.
- In those who are poorly peg/ribavirin responsive, an additional stopping rule of $<10^3$ HCV RNA reduction at Week 8 seems to help minimize the likelihood of reducing resistance-associated variants.
- Additional data in special populations, including HIV/Hepatitis C coinfected, those with cirrhosis, and those with Hepatitis C recurrence after orthotopic liver transplant are required to assess the efficacy of boceprevir in these populations.

In May 2011, the direct acting antiviral therapies boceprevir and telaprevir, both NS3/NS4 protease inhibitors, were approved for the treatment of genotype I Hepatitis C in combination with peginterferon and ribavirin (PR). Boceprevir when added with PR, significantly improved sustained response (SVR) rates in the treatment of genotype I treatment-naïve patients and those who had failed previous therapy. This approval was based on 2 large registration trials. The Sprint 2 trial examined the efficacy of boceprevir in treatment-naïve patients, whereas the Respond 2 trial examined the efficacy of boceprevir therapy in partial responders and relapsers to previous PR therapy. This review examines the current treatment paradigm of boceprevir-based treatment

Dr Paul Kwo has received contracted research funding from Abbott, Bayer, Bristol Myers Squibb, Glaxo Smith Kline, Gilead, Merck, Roche, and Vertex, served on advisory boards for Abbott, Bristol Myers Squibb, Gilead, Merck, Novartis, Vertex; he also received fees for Non-CME/CE services directly from Bristol Myers Squibb, Merck, and Vertex.
Gastroenterology/Hepatology Division, Indiana University School of Medicine, 975 West Walnut, IB 327, Indianapolis, IN 46202-5121, USA
E-mail address: pkwo@iupui.edu

of chronic hepatitis C, examining treatment paradigms, predictors of response, futility rules, as well as preliminary results from studies examining boceprevir efficacy in additional populations.

The current treatment recommendations for boceprevir in combination with peginterferon and ribavirin are derived from the large Phase 3 Sprint 2 and Respond 2 studies. In the Sprint 2 study, a total of 938 nonblack and 159 black patients were treated with peginterferon alfa-2b and ribavirin (PR) or boceprevir plus peginterferon and ribavirin in a response-guided paradigm for a fixed duration of 44 weeks.[1] The control group received the previous standard of care PR for 48 weeks (Group 1). Group 2 received boceprevir plus PR for 24 weeks in a response-guided paradigm in combination with boceprevir after a 4-week lead-in of PR, with those with having detectable HCV RNA levels between Week 8 and 24 receiving an additional 20 weeks of PR for a total of 48 weeks. The third group received fixed duration boceprevir for 44 weeks with peginterferon and ribavirin after a 4-week PR lead-in. In the nonblack cohort, boceprevir in the response-guided arm led to an overall SVR rate of 67%, which was virtually identical to the 68% SVR rate seen in the group with fixed duration boceprevir with peginterferon and ribavirin treatment. Both were statistically higher than the PR control group of 40%. In the black cohort, which had the same study design, the SVR rate in both the fixed and response-guided paradigm arms were superior to PR control (53% and 42% vs 23% respectively), although numerically higher SVR rates were seen with fixed duration boceprevir 44 weeks with peginterferon and ribavirin in this cohort. Moreover, the 4-week PR lead-in viral decline was an important tool in predicting the SVR rate, with those having a greater than 1 log reduction of the SVR rate experiencing an 82% overall SVR rate with boceprevir addition, regardless of response-guided or fixed duration boceprevir treatment. In the black cohort, SVR rates were also higher, with greater than 1 log decline from baseline during the 4 weeks of peginterferon and ribavirin treatment at 67% and 61%, respectively. After the Food and Drug Administration review, boceprevir was approved for a response-guided paradigm in noncirrhotic individuals and those who had greater than 1 log reduction during the 4-week peg/ribavirin lead-in. These individuals could receive a 4-week peg/ribavirin lead-in, followed by 24 weeks of peginterferon and ribavirin with boceprevir in those who are at Treatment Week 8 to 24 undetectable, truncation of therapy at 28 weeks is appropriate. Those with detectable virus at Week 8 and who clear virus by Week 24 receive 32 weeks of boceprevir and PR and then a 12-week tail of PR. In the PR poorly responsive individuals (those with <1 log reduction during the lead-in) and those with cirrhosis, 44 weeks of boceprevir with PR is provided. Treatment week futility rules were set as HCV RNA level greater than 100 IU/mL at Week 12 or Week 24 detectable levels of HCV RNA, during which all therapy should be discontinued because SVR will not occur, to minimize the development of resistance-associated variants (RAVs).

With the use of boceprevir for genotype 1 hepatitis C, all subjects receive a 4-week PR lead-in. The 4-week peg/ribavirin lead-in initially was examined in the Sprint 1 study, in which it was hypothesized that steady state levels of peginterferon and ribavirin achieved after 4 weeks would minimize the development of RAVs and improve SVR rates.[2] No statistically significant difference in SVR rates were noted in the Sprint 1 study between lead-in and non–lead-in groups, although the 4-week peg/ribavirin lead-in provided prognostic information about the opportunity to achieve SVR. At present, the lead-in should be used as a tool that allows the assessment of the patient's ability to tolerate the backbone PR before the addition of a direct-acting antiviral therapy.

In those who have failed peginterferon and ribavirin treatment, the treatment paradigm is based on the large Respond 2 study.[3] Patients again were randomized into 3 groups. Treatment Group 1 was the control group and received 48 weeks of PR.

Group 2 received response-guided therapy (RGT) with boceprevir for 32 weeks with those who cleared virus between Weeks 8 and 24 receiving a total of 32 weeks of therapy and those with a detectable levels of HCV RNA at Week 8 who clear virus by Week 24 receiving a total of 48 weeks of therapy, with an additional 12 week peginterferon and ribavirin after the 32 weeks of triple therapy. Group 3 received 44 weeks of boceprevir, peginterferon, and ribavirin after the lead-in 4-week peg/ribavirin lead-in (fixed). In this study, relapsers and partial responders (>2 log HCV RNA reduction with peginterferon and ribavirin after Week 12 but never undetected) were enrolled. Null responders specifically were excluded. An overall SVR rate of 59% in the response-guided arm and a 66% SVR rate in the fixed-duration boceprevir group was observed, statistically higher than the 21% SVR seen in the peginterferon/ribavirin lead treatment control. Partial relapsers had higher SVR rates, 69% (RGT) and 75% (fixed), compared with PR control at 29%. Partial responders had higher SVR rates with fixed duration therapy (52% vs 7% in the PR control) than RGT (40%). Thus, the treatment paradigm for nonresponders includes a total of 32 weeks of boceprevir after a 4-week peg/ribavirin lead-in, with those having HCV RNA treatment at Week 8 and 24 undetectable, truncating all therapy at Week 36, which differs from those who are naïve in whom treatment is truncated at week 28 (**Fig. 1**). Those with detectable levels of HCV RNA at treatment Week 8 but with undetectable levels at treatment Week 24 complete a total of 48 weeks of therapy with the PR tail of 12 weeks after the 32 weeks of triple therapy (**Fig. 2**). Similar to naïve patients, those who are cirrhotic and those who are poorly responsive (<1 log reduction with PR lead in) receive 48 weeks of therapy with 44 weeks of triple therapy after the peg/ribavirin lead-in. Futility rules are identical to those who are treatment naïve individuals with an HCV RNA level greater than 100 IU/mL at Week 12, or detectable HCV RNA level at treatment Week 24 also lead to truncation of therapy.

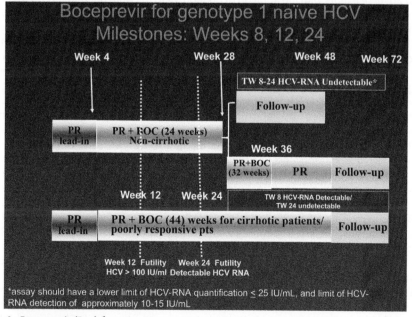

Fig. 1. Boceprevir (Boc) for genotype 1 naïve patients. Key treatment time points are treatment weeks (TW) 8, 12, and 24.

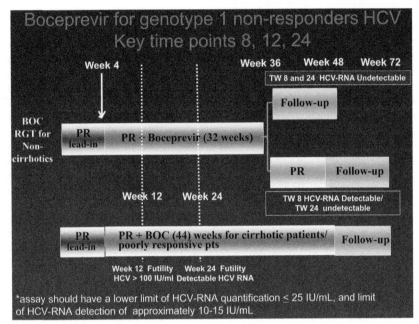

Fig. 2. Boceprevir (Boc) for genotype 1 nonresponders. Key treatment time points are treatment weeks (TW) 8, 12, and 24.

ROLE OF ANEMIA

New adverse events with the addition of boceprevir to PR were not detected. Two side effects, anemia and dysgeusia, were noted at higher rates in the boceprevir-containing regimens compared with the peginterferon/ribavirin control group. In both the Sprint 2 and Respond 2 trials, erythropoietin was allowed at investigator discretion to help manage anemia. Anemia has been a well-known complication in the treatment of Hepatitis C related to the ribavirin-related hemolysis and peginterferon-related bone marrow suppression. In those receiving therapy for Hepatitis C with peginterferon and ribavirin, up to 30% of individuals experience anemia.[4,5] Boceprevir contributes an approximate one additional 1 g hemoglobin decline, although anemia as a serious adverse event was rarely reported in the registration trials (1%). The mechanism of anemia is thought to be the result of bone marrow suppressive effect associated with boceprevir and not because of additional red blood cell hemolysis. In the Sprint 2 study, in the boceprevir-containing regimen, 73% of individuals in the response-guided boceprevir arm and 74% of individuals in the fixed duration boceprevir arm experienced Grade 1 or 2 anemia toxicities (hemoglobin reduction to 8 g/dL) versus a total of 43% in the PR control. Grade 3 or higher anemia (hemoglobin to <6.5 g/dL) was rare in the control as well as the boceprevir containing arms (2%–3%). A retrospective analysis of the Sprint 1 and Sprint 2 studies suggested that regardless of anemia management strategy (erythropoietin alone, ribavirin dose reduction alone, both or neither) that SVR rates were similar in the Sprint 2 and Respond 2 studies.[6]

To address the optimal management of anemia in boceprevir-treated individuals, a recent study evaluated in a randomized trial ribavirin dose reduction versus erythropoietin for anemia management in treatment naïve patients receiving boceprevir plus peginterferon and ribavirin, the preliminary results of which have been presented.[7] In this study, patients who developed anemia were randomized to receive either ribavirin dose reduction or initiation of erythropoietin without ribavirin dose reduction. A secondary anemia strategy could also be used, including erythropoietin, ribavirin dose reduction, or transfusion. The overall SVR rate was 63% and the anemia cohort achieved an overall SVR rate of 71.2% (356/500). When the randomized arms were compared, identical SVR rates were observed with dose reduction and erythropoietin initiation of 71% in both arms. The preliminary results from this large study suggest that ribavirin dose reduction should be the initial treatment strategy for the adverse event for the additional anemia associated with boceprevir addition to peginterferon and ribavirin.

PREDICTORS OF RESPONSE TO BOCEPREVIR

Many of the predictor factors that predict a response to boceprevir in combination with peginterferon and ribavirin for genotype I Hepatitis C are similar to the predictors of response with peginterferon and ribavirin therapy. Before the introduction of NS3/NS4 protease inhibitor addition to PR, low viral load, younger age, lack of insulin resistance adherence, rapid virologic response, ribavirin dose administration, black race, interleukin (IL) 28B genotype, and anemia were important predictive factors of response.[8] The addition of direct-acting antiviral agents, such as boceprevir, has introduced additional predictors including genotype 1a/1b, statin use, and on-treatment response to the peginterferon/ribavirin lead-in.

The pretreatment predictors of response for boceprevir-based therapy are comparable to those with PR therapy. In the Sprint 2 study, those of nonblack race achieved the highest SVR rates. Fixed-duration boceprevir treatment in the black cohort was associated with the highest SVR (53% compared with 23%), reflecting the poor PR responsiveness of this group. Similar to PR therapy, age also was associated with numerically higher SVR rates, those who are aged 40 years and younger achieving higher SVR rates with boceprevir-based therapy of 69% (fixed) and 73% (RGT) compared with 65% (fixed) and 64% (RGT) in those older than 40 years. However, it seemed that the addition of boceprevir improved the SVR rates to a greater numeric degree in those older than 40 years compared with those in the peg/ribavirin control (65% and 64% vs 34% in PR controls). Viral levels also were associated with SVR, with those with low viral levels (<800,000 IU/mL) with boceprevir-based therapy achieving high SVR rates of 85% and 76% compared with those with >800,000 I.U. achieving SVR rates of 63% and 61%. Historically, genotype I has been associated with lower SVR rates; however, a few data to differentiate genotype 1a and 1b were available. A large randomized trial comparing peginterferon alfa-2b with peginterferon alfa-2a showed no difference in the overall SVR rates.[8] However, the addition of boceprevir to PR was associated with higher SVR rates in the genotype 1b cohort compared with the genotype 1a cohort.In the boceprevir-containing regimens, genotype 1b was associated with higher SVR rates of 70% and 66% in the fixed duration and response-guided arm compared with 63% and 59% in genotype 1a. In the PR control, genotype 1b was also associated with a higher SVR rate of 40% compared with that of 35% in genotype 1a. However, the incremental improvement in SVR remained comparable. The reasons for the difference in SVR rates are unclear. Previous studies have suggested that genotype 1b may indeed be associated with a more favorable SVR rate than genotype 1a with peginterferon and ribavirin without direct-acting antiviral agents, although a large study disputed this.[8–10] Moreover, the initial HCV replicons were developed in genotype 1b models; and, thus, initial drug selection was in genotype 1b replicon variants.[11] Moreover, the number of mutations required to develop resistance for genotype 1b is greater than that for 1a in those receiving boceprevir.[12]

The role of hepatic fibrosis is also important because the lack of fibrosis predicts SVR with PR-based therapy.[8] In the control group, in Sprint 2 treatment-naïve individuals, those with F0 to F2 had identical SVR rates to those with F3/F4 (38% in each group), although the cohort in the F3/F4 had a small sample size (9/34). The addition of boceprevir was associated with an approximately 30% improvement in SVR rate in those with F0 to F2 over PR control (38%–67%) in both boceprevir-containing regimens versus a lower numeric improvement in SVR rate in the F3/F4 cohort of 38% to 52% in the fixed-duration arm boceprevir and 38% to 41% in F3/F4 with RGT arm. These results suggest that fixed-duration boceprevir therapy is preferred in those with cirrhosis. An additional pretreatment factor associated with boceprevir, in addition to peginterferon and ribavirin, was the influence of statin use on SVR. Although the sample size is small, those who used statins with boceprevir therapy experienced high SVR rates of 86% and 67%. The potential association of statin use with SVR is not clear. The Hepatitis C virus forms lipoviral particles that represent the primary form of Hepatitis C within the circulation. The low-density lipoprotein receptor is thought to be key in binding and entry of the virus into the hepatocyte, which may explain the statin results.[13] Moreover, statins seem to have intrinsic antiviral properties with antiviral activities being demonstrated in HIV virus, respiratory syncytial virus, and Hepatitis C virus. However, there are significant drug-drug interactions with boceprevir as well as telaprevir, and although certain statins are certainly safe with boceprevir, further data will be required before statin use could definitively be used to improve SVR rates.

The genetic polymorphism IL28B is the strongest pretreatment predictor of response.[14] A retrospective analyses from the large Sprint 2 and Respond 2 databases demonstrates that IL28B genotype also predicts response in those treated with boceprevir and PR. In a recent report, 62% of individuals consented to IL28B genomic testing (653/1048).[15] Overall SVR rates in IL28BCC (favorable groups) were comparable across the boceprevir-containing arms compared with the peg/ribavirin arm. However, in the more difficult to treat patients with the IL-28B CT and IL-28B TT groups who have less PR responsiveness, the addition of boceprevir was associated with markedly higher SVR rates compared with those in the PR control group (PR control 28% and 27% vs 65%–71% in IL28B CT and 55%–59% in IL28B TT groups). Although these results are incomplete datasets based on retrospective analyses, this preliminary evidence suggests that boceprevir addition to PR is a substantial predictor in successful therapy with genotype I and may predict the short duration of therapy (28 weeks) in those with favorable IL28B CC genotype.

However, on-treatment factors have been shown to be the most powerful predictors of SVR in those receiving. In a recent multivariate analysis, the 4-week PR lead-in response (>1 log reduction from baseline) was the most powerful predictor of SVR when incorporated in a mulitvariate model that included pretreatment and on-treatment factors.[15] As previously discussed, anemia was also identified as a significant factor for attaining SVR and boceprevir-based therapies similar to what is seen in peginterferon/ribavirin-based therapy.

FUTILITY RULES

In the era of direct-acting antiviral agents, futility rules must be adhered to, given the need to reduce the risk of emergence of RAVs. Based on a large Phase 2 and 3 boceprevir trials, the existing futility rules, including an HCV RNA of 100 IU/mL or more at Week 12 of therapy (after 8 weeks of boceprevir and 12 weeks of triple therapy) or detectable HCV RNA levels at Week 24. An additional stopping rule has been suggested in individuals who are poor responders to the peginterferon/ribavirin lead-in. In this subanalysis from the Sprint 2 and Respond 2 studies, those who were poorly PR responsive (<1 log reduction in the lead-in) with less than 10^3 (1000-fold) reduction after Treatment Week 8 (4 weeks of boceprevir) had no opportunity to achieve SVR.[16] Thus in poor PR responders, although not in the boceprevir label, this important stopping rule should be strongly considered by clinicians who treat those who are poorly peg/ribavirin responsive.

NULL RESPONDERS

The large Phase 3 Respond 2 study enrolled partial responders and relapsers to a 12-week course of peginterferon and ribavirin. However, preliminary data from the Provide study have been presented, suggesting that well-defined null responders may also be successfully treated with boceprevir-based therapy.[17] In this study, patients who had in received peginterferon and ribavirin as control and failed to achieve SVR were enrolled to receive open label 4-week peg/ribavirin lead-in, followed by the administration of boceprevir 800 mg 3 times a day with ribavirin 600 to 1400 mg a day. In this study, 52/168 individuals were null responders with less than 2 log reduction at Week 12 with PCR, 26/168 (15%) were prior relapsers, and 35% (85/168) were prior partial responders. Although final results are not available, the interim reports suggest that null responders will have a high SVR rate, with 19 of 47 (40%) null responders achieving SVR compared with 53 out of 78 (68%) SVR in partial responders. Relapse rates were low at 14% and 15%, respectively. The final results from this prospective cohort are awaited. However, preliminary report suggests that boceprevir addition to peginterferon and ribavirin may be used as therapy in well-defined null responders, in addition to those with partial response or relapse. However, the effect on null responders with cirrhosis remains unknown. At present, boceprevir is not Food and Drug Administration approved for null responders.

THE ROLE OF BOCEPREVIR IN COINFECTED INDIVIDUALS

There have been no large randomized trials to date in those who are HIV/Hepatitis C coinfected. Previous studies with peginterferon and ribavirin have demonstrated lower SVR rates in HIV/Hepatitis C coinfected compared with historical controls. Moreover, the drug-drug interactions with antiretroviral therapies theoretically may be problematic. A preliminary report demonstrates that boceprevir addition to peginterferon and ribavirin in genotype 1 Hepatitis C infected individuals is feasible.[18] In this study, genotype I infected individuals with HIV infection under good control (<50 copies/mL on antiretroviral therapy and CD4 count >200 cells/mm^3) were enrolled to receive peginterferon and ribavirin for 4 weeks, followed by boceprevir addition. A control group of 48 weeks of peginterferon and ribavirin were included. In this cohort, 98 individuals were enrolled with a mean age of 44 years. Of note, decompensated cirrhotics were excluded, as were the use of several antiretroviral therapies (zidovudine, didanosine, stavudine, efavirenz, etravirine, and nevirapine). In this cohort, 64 individuals received boceprevir-based therapy and 34 individuals received peginterferon and ribavirin therapy. A preliminary SVR rate of 61% was noted in the boceprevir-containing regimens compared with a 27% SVR rate in those treated with peginterferon and ribavirin. The number of serious adverse events was comparable in the cohorts and, in particular, hematologic events were similar, other than a higher use of erythropoietin in the boceprevir cohort. HIV breakthroughs did occur in 3 of 64 individuals receiving boceprevir-based therapy and 4 of 34 individuals in the control group. The final SVR results are eagerly awaited.

COST-EFFECTIVENESS OF BOCEPREVIR WITH PEGINTERFERON AND RIBAVIRIN

Two preliminary reports have suggested that boceprevir, in addition to peginterferon and ribavirin, are cost-effective therapies in naïve patients and those with prior nonresponse to peginterferon and ribavirin treatment. In one report, a Markov model was designed based on the US costs to determine whether or not boceprevir addition to PR could improve SVR in a cost-effective manner, with assumptions of a daily cost of peginterferon alfa-2b of $84, ribavirin of $44, boceprevir $157, monitoring costs $64, and the cost of treating anemia at $125.[19] Treatment with boceprevir in both response-guided paradigm and fixed-duration boceprevir were examined. Treatment with boceprevir in a response-guided paradigm was predicted to result in up to 38% fewer cases of decompensation, hepatocellular carcinoma, orthotopic liver transplant, or liver-related death compared with treatment with peginterferon and ribavirin. Treatment with fixed duration was expected to result in 43% fewer cases of decompensated liver disease, hepatoma, transplant, or liver-related death. Using a cost-effectiveness acceptability curve, at a threshold of $50,000, boceprevir added to peginterferon and ribavirin in a response-guided paradigm was effective at a $50,000 willingness to pay per additional quality of life year, and fixed duration boceprevir was cost-effective at a threshold of $100,000. In nonresponders, similar findings were noted with boceprevir-based regimens being cost-effective compared with nonresponders (modeled on relapsers ad partial responders) at similar thresholds of $50,000 for RGT and $100,000 for fixed duration boceprevir.[20] A recent European study noted that boceprevir was cost-effective for IL28B TT infected individuals, compared with PR.[21] To date, there are no cost-effectiveness studies in null responders for the use of boceprevir.

BOCEPREVIR IN ADVANCED FIBROSIS AND POSTORTHOTOPIC LIVER TRANSPLANT

In the treatment of those with cirrhosis, preliminary data come from France, where the French compassionate use of protease inhibitors in cirrhotics (CUPIC cohort) examined genotype I individuals with compensated cirrhosis (Child Pugh A) who were relapsers and partial responders to previous PR.[22] In this cohort, null responders were excluded. In a recent interim analysis of Week 16, virologic results and safety data were reported. In this cohort, 159 individuals had received boceprevir-based therapy. Twenty-six percent of the cohort had criteria that would have excluded them from the Phase 3 trial Respond 2. However, most individuals were Child A infected individuals. In the 159 individuals with advanced fibrosis, 38.4% of individuals experienced severe adverse effects, with 2 out of 159 dying because of a pulmonary infection and the others dying because of sepsis. Not surprisingly, anemia was problematic, with 22.6% of the cohort experiencing Grade 2 anemia and 10% experiencing Grade 3 to 4 anemia (hemoglobin <8 g/dL). Erythropoietin use, not surprisingly, was high at 66% of the cohort and 11% of individuals (17 out 159 received blood transfusions). Efficacy rates through Week 16 were reported, with 61% of individuals clearing virus by Week 16. Additional results will be reported at future meetings; however, these preliminary results demonstrate that severe anemia will be problematic in those with advanced liver disease, although on-treatment virologic clearance rates seem to be high with boceprevir addition to PR. The French experience with boceprevir addition to PR for severe Hepatitis C recurrence after liver transplantation was also reported.[23] Patients who received boceprevir were given a 4-week peg/ribavirin lead-in, followed by addition of 800 mg of boceprevir three times a day. Thus far, 70 patients have completed through Week 8 of boceprevir, with 56% of individuals on boceprevir by Week 8 having undetectable HCV RNA levels. Infections, blood transfusion, anemia, and thrombocytopenia were all noted, again attributing to the high rate of SAEs. Additional follow-up of this cohort will be reported.

In conclusion, the addition of boceprevir to peginterferon and ribavirin has improved SVR rates markedly. Boceprevir is effective in treatment naïve, relapsers, partial responders, and null responders. Those with advanced fibrosis require 44 weeks of boceprevir therapy after a 4-week peg/ribavirin lead-in. The main side effect with boceprevir is anemia and ribavirin dose reduction is an effective strategy. In those who are poorly peg/ribavirin responsive to peg/ribavirin treatment, an additional stopping rule of less than 10^3 HCV RNA reduction at Week 8 seems to help minimize the likelihood of reducing RAVs. Special populations, including HIV/Hepatitis C coinfected, those with cirrhosis, and those with Hepatitis C recurrence after orthotopic liver transplant, all may benefit from boceprevir-based therapy. Further follow-up in these cohorts will be required.

REFERENCES

1. Poordad F, McCone J Jr, Bacon BR, et al. Boceprevir for untreated chronic HCV genotype 1 infection. N Engl J Med 2011;364:1195–206.
2. Kwo PY, Lawitz EJ, McCone J, et al. Efficacy of boceprevir, an NS3 protease inhibitor, in combination with peginterferon alfa-2b and ribavirin in treatment-naive patients with genotype 1 hepatitis C infection (SPRINT-1): an open-label, randomised, multicentre phase 2 trial. Lancet 2010;376:705–16.
3. Bacon BR, Gordon SC, Lawitz E, et al. Boceprevir for previously treated chronic HCV genotype 1 infection. N Engl J Med 2011;364:1207–17.
4. Shiffman ML, Salvatore J, Hubbard S, et al. Treatment of chronic hepatitis C virus genotype 1 with peginterferon, ribavirin, and epoetin alpha. Hepatology 2007;46: 371–9.
5. Sulkowski MS, Shiffman ML, Afdhal NH, et al. Hepatitis C virus treatment-related anemia is associated with higher sustained virologic response rate. Gastroenterology 2010;139:1602–11, 11 e1.
6. Sulkowski MS, Poordad F, Manns MP, et al. Anemia during treatment with peginterferon alfa-2b/ ribavirin with or without boceprevir is associated with higher SVR rates: analysis of previously untreated and previous-treatment-failure patients. J Hepatol 2011;54:S194–5.
7. Poordad FF, Lawitz EJ, Reddy KR, et al. 1419 A randomized trial comparing ribavirin dose reduction versus erythropoietin for anemia management in previously untreated patients with chronic hepatitis C receiving boceprevir plus peginterferon/ribavirin. J Hepatol 2012;56:S559.
8. McHutchison JG, Lawitz EJ, Shiffman ML, et al. Peginterferon alfa-2b or alfa-2a with ribavirin for treatment of hepatitis C infection. N Engl J Med 2009;361:580–93.
9. Nicot F, Alric L, Barange K, et al. Influence of HCV genotype 1 subtypes on the virus response to PEG interferon alpha-2a plus ribavirin therapy. J Med Virol 2011;83:437–44.
10. Legrand-Abravanel F, Colson P, Leguillou-Guillemette H, et al. Influence of the HCV subtype on the virological response to pegylated interferon and ribavirin therapy. J Med Virol 2009;81:2029–35.
11. Lohmann V, Korner F, Koch J, et al. Replication of subgenomic hepatitis C virus RNAs in a hepatoma cell line. Science 1999;285:110–3.

12. Kwo PY, Vinayek R. The therapeutic approaches for hepatitis C virus: protease inhibitors and polymerase inhibitors. Gut Liver 2011;5:406–17.
13. Rao GA, Pandya PK. Statin therapy improves sustained virologic response among diabetic patients with chronic hepatitis C. Gastroenterology 2011;140: 144–52.
14. Thompson AJ, Muir AJ, Sulkowski MS, et al. Interleukin-28B polymorphism improves viral kinetics and is the strongest pretreatment predictor of sustained virologic response in genotype 1 hepatitis C virus. Gastroenterology 2010;139. 120–129.e18.
15. Poordad F, Bronowicki JP, Gordon SC, et al. Factors that predict response of patients with hepatitis C virus infection to boceprevir. Gastroenterology 2012; 43(3). 608–618.e5.
16. Bruce R, Bacon SB, Eugene R. Predictors of sustained virologic response (SVR) among poor interferon (IFN) responders when boceprevir (BOC) is added to peginterferon alfa-2b/ribavirin (PR) [abstract 33]. Hepatology 2011;54:76A.
17. Bronowicki JP, Davis M, Flamm S, et al. 11 Sustained virologic response (SVR) in prior peginterferon/ribavirin (PR) treatment failures after retreatment with boceprevir (BOC) -+-PR: the provide study interim results. J Hepatol 2012;56:S6.
18. Mallolas J, SP, Rivero A, et al. Boceprevir plus peginterferon/ribavirin for the treatment of HCV/HIV co-infected patients: end of treatment (week 48) interim results. J Hepatol 2012;S22.
19. Ferrante SA, JC, Elbasha E, et al. A US-based cost-effectiveness analysis of boceprevir-based regimens in previously untreated adult subjects with chronic hepatitis C genotype 1. Hepatology 2011;54:199A.
20. Chhatwal J, Ferrante SA, Dasbach EJ, et al. Cost-effectiveness of boceprevir use in patients with chronic hepatitis C genotype-1 who failed prior treatment with peginterferon/Ribavirin. Hepatology 2011;54:200A.
21. Cammà C, Petta S, Enea M, et al. Cost-effectiveness of boceprevir or telaprevir for untreated patients with genotype 1 chronic hepatitis C. Hepatology 2012; 56(3):850–60.
22. Hezode C, Dorival C, Zoulim F, et al. 8 Safety of telaprevir or boceprevir in combination with peginterferon alfa/ribavirin, in cirrhotic non responders. First results of the French early access program. (ANRS CO20-CUPIC). J Hepatol 2012;56:S4.
23. Coilly A, BR, Botta-Fridlund D, et al. Efficacy and safety of protease inhibitors for severe hepatitis C recurrence after liver transplantation: a first multicenter experience. J Hepatol 2012;56:S21, 47A.

Management of the Transplant Recipient with Chronic Hepatitis C

James R. Burton Jr, MD, Gregory T. Everson, MD*

KEYWORDS

- Telaprevir • Boceprevir • Transplant • Hepatitis C virus

KEY POINTS

- Rapid advances in new drug therapy to treat the recurrence of infection with the hepatitis C virus promise to improve overall outcomes, reduce side effects, shorten treatment duration, simplify treatment regimens, and lower risk for drug-drug interactions.
- The emerging data suggest that current triple therapy should be used with caution by experienced clinicians in liver centers and with very close monitoring of side effects and adverse events.
- Drug-drug interactions are common and potentially dangerous. The transplant hepatologist must be prepared to lower doses of immunosuppressive medications and closely monitor drug levels at the onset of triple therapy. After stopping telaprevir or boceprevir, doses of immunosuppressive medications must be increased and drug levels closely monitored.
- The hope of future treatments includes pangenotype coverage, reduced side effects, lack of bone marrow suppression, elimination of drug-drug interactions, and ultimately Food and Drug Administration–approved indications for use of antiviral treatment before and after liver transplantation.
- Transplant hepatologists, pharmaceutical partners, and liver recipients should work together to push up the timelines.

Recurrence of infection with the hepatitis C virus (HCV) after liver transplantation is associated with accelerated graft loss and diminished patient survival, and treatment options are limited.[1,2] Based on recent OPTN data, more than one-third of the potential recipients on the waiting list for liver transplantation in the United States are infected with HCV. The percentage of patients receiving transplants who are infected with HCV may be even higher—primarily due to the development of hepatocellular carcinoma before listing or while waiting. For example, in our own program in Colorado, 53% of the patients with highest Model for End-Stage Liver Disease (MELD) scores, representing the patients likely to be transplanted, are infected with HCV and two-thirds of these HCV patients have MELD upgrade for hepatocellular

Department of Medicine, University of Colorado Denver, 1635 Aurora Court, B-154, Aurora, CO 80045, USA
* Corresponding author.
E-mail address: greg.everson@ucdenver.edu

Clin Liver Dis 17 (2013) 73–91
http://dx.doi.org/10.1016/j.cld.2012.09.013
1089-3261/13/$ – see front matter © 2013 Published by Elsevier Inc.

liver.theclinics.com

carcinoma. Given the high proportion of liver recipients infected with HCV and its adverse effects on graft and patient survival, treatment and eradication of HCV before or after transplantation are a high priority for transplant hepatologists.

The main goal of treating the transplant recipient infected with HCV is to achieve sustained viral response (SVR)—undetectable HCV RNA 12 weeks or more after the end of treatment. SVR preserves graft function, improves graft survival, and improves both patient outcome and patient survival.[3,4] However, the effectiveness of current antiviral treatment of transplant recipients is limited by poor tolerability and suboptimal cure rates.

Today's preferred antiviral treatments for HCV are based on HCV genotype (GT): peginterferon/ribavirin (PEG/RBV) plus either telaprevir or boceprevir (triple therapy, TT) for GT 1,[5–9] and PEG/RBV alone for non-1 HCV genotypes.[10–12] Despite the widespread use of PEG/RBV and emerging experience with TT, there have been few randomized, placebo-controlled trials in liver recipients. Nearly all published results represent single-center experiences, which are subject to significant differences in the selection of patients and bias in reporting and interpreting results.

In this review, the authors present cases, discuss treatment strategies, define the current experience with both PEG/RBV and TT, and speculate on the potential improvement in rates of SVR with future regimens using direct-acting antivirals.

CAVEAT: TT is not FDA-approved for use before, during, or after liver transplantation—its use in this setting is "OFF-LABEL."

STRATEGY 1: PRETRANSPLANT TREATMENT

The main goal of pretransplant treatment with antiviral therapy is to prevent the recurrence of HCV infection in the allograft (posttransplant viral response [pTVR]), thereby improving graft and patient outcomes.[13,14] However, waiting list patients with cirrhosis, particularly those with decompensation and high MELD scores, may not tolerate interferon-based treatment and are prone to serious complications including infection, hepatic failure, and even death. For these reasons, candidacy for pretransplant therapy with interferon-based regimens is limited to the patient who is either

- A potential recipient of a graft from a living donor, or
- A potential recipient with MELD upgrade for hepatocellular carcinoma (HCC).

These 2 groups of recipients are characterized by lower disease-defined MELD score, less hepatic impairment, and potentially greater tolerability of PEG/RBV.

Case 1: Treating a Patient Prior to Liver Transplantation

A 44-year-old patient with cirrhosis due to HCV developed a 3.1-cm HCC. Except for the HCC, his clinical course was stable without variceal bleeding, ascites, or hepatic encephalopathy. MELD score, based on bilirubin, international normalized ratio (INR), and creatinine, was 9. He was listed for liver transplantation, received a MELD upgrade to 22, and was referred for transarterial chemoembolization of the HCC. The patient stated that 2 of his family members are considering the option of living donation.

Laboratory evaluation included HCV genotype 1a, HCV RNA level 2,100,000 IU/mL, IL28b genotype CT, white blood cell count (WBC) 3200/μL, hemoglobin 12.5 g/dL, and platelet count 105,000/μL.

The patient was interested in treatment to prevent the recurrence of HCV infection in his transplanted liver.

This case represents the ideal candidate for consideration of pretransplant treatment using interferon-based antiviral therapy. The characteristics that favor successful treatment are as follows:

- MELD upgrade for HCC
- Potential candidacy for LDLT
- Low MELD by bilirubin, INR, and creatinine
- No clinical complications of cirrhosis
- Potential to define the duration of antiviral treatment

Sensitivity to interferon is another variable that favors SVR. In treatment-naïve patients, IL28b polymorphism CC (vs CT or TT) is the strongest single predictor of SVR.[15,16] In treatment-experienced patients, the response to the prior course of PEG/RBV also defines likelihood of SVR in response to retreatment with TT (relapse > partial > null).[7]

Case 1 (Continued)

One question was whether to use PEG/RBV alone or TT. The authors elected to use TT due to the higher SVR, compared with PEG/RBV, in patients with compensated cirrhosis.

This patient is infected with HCV genotype 1a, an HCV genotype that can be treated with either PEG/RBV or TT. The authors chose TT based on the results of the ADVANCE, ILLUMINATE, and SPRINT-2 studies.

Study	Rates of SVR in Cirrhosis	
	PEG/RBV	Triple Therapy
ADVANCE[5]	33%	62%
ILLUMINATE[6]	ND	63%
SPRINT-2[8]	38%	52%

From the SVR perspective, TT is likely a better option. However, telaprevir and boceprevir add additional side effects, particularly anemia, that diminish the tolerability of the regimen. Patients with cirrhosis are already prone to anemia and other cytopenias, which worsen under PEG/RBV treatment, and anemia is further exacerbated by the addition of either telaprevir or boceprevir.

Early experience indicates that TT does increase viral response in cirrhosis, but anemia is severe, poorly responsive to erythropoietin analog (EPO), and often requires blood transfusion. The ANRS-CUPIC study compared on-treatment outcomes with either telaprevir-based (N = 169) or boceprevir-based (N = 138) TT in patients with cirrhosis who relapsed or had a partial response during a prior course of treatment with PEG/RBV.[17] At week 12 of TT, 71% of boceprevir-based and 86% of telaprevir-based treatment had undetectable HCV RNA. Treatment was discontinued prematurely in 26% because of side effects; 15% of patients had serious adverse events, and 2% of patients died. Anemia was a major management issue.

Everson and Burton evaluated 37 patients with cirrhosis that were treated with TT, 13 of whom were listed for transplantation, and 27 of these were treatment-experienced (null 15, partial 2, relapse 10) (Everson GT, unpublished data, presented at American Transplant Congress 2012.). By week 4, 85% had HCV RNA <1000 IU/mL.

Forty-three percent achieved an extended rapid viral response (HCV RNA <18 IU/mL (LOD) from weeks 4 through 12) and our projected rate for SVR is 50%. Anemia was a main adverse event requiring ribavirin dose reduction, EPO, or blood transfusions in 75% of cases.

Case 1 (Continued)

HCV RNA became undetectable after week 4 of TT and remained undetectable during treatment. Anemia was managed by ribavirin dose reduction to 600 mg/d, EPO, and 1 transfusion of 2 U of packed red blood cells (RBCs). At week 36 of a planned 48 weeks of treatment (12 weeks telaprevir/PEG/RBV followed by 36 weeks of PEG/RBV), a liver transplant was performed and antiviral therapy was stopped. Tumor stage was T1N0M0. Twelve weeks after liver transplantation, HCV RNA has remained undetectable.

Our patient achieved an extended rapid viral response (eRVR, undetectable HCV RNA from weeks 4 through 12) despite cirrhosis, high viral load, and GT 1a infection. Based on the ILLUMINATE study, noncirrhotic patients who achieve eRVR may stop telaprevir-based TT at week 24.[6] However, the Food and Drug Administration recommends continuing the PEG/RBV to week 48 in patients with cirrhosis with eRVR, even though this issue has not undergone formal study. The authors had planned for 48 weeks, but a liver came available at week 36 of treatment and the authors proceeded with the transplant. As of 12 weeks posttransplant, the patient shows no recurrence of HCV and it is hopeful that he is cured—not only of his HCV infection but also HCC!

In contrast to the minimal information regarding use of TT in patients with cirrhosis or those on the waiting list, there are several published series of single-center experience with the use of PEG/RBV in this setting.[18–26] Rates of pTVR have ranged from 20% to 28% but side effects were common and serious, even life-threatening, complications occurred (**Table 1**).

There is 1 published randomized controlled trial of PEG/RBV treatment to prevent the recurrence of HCV after liver transplantation.[27] Centers within the Adult-to-Adult Living Donor Liver Transplantation Cohort Study enrolled HCV patients who were listed for liver transplantation, with either potential living donors or MELD upgrade for hepatocellular carcinoma. Patients with HCV GT 1/4/6 (n = 44/2/1) were randomized 2:1 to treatment or untreated control; patients with HCV GT 2/3 were assigned to treatment.

Table 1			
Pretransplant treatment to prevent posttransplant recurrence			
Author	**Patients, N**	**RNA Negative Day of LTx**	**pTVR**
Carrion[21]	51	29%	20%
Everson[26]	47	32%	26%
Forns[23]	30	30%	20%
Thomas[25]	20	60%	20%
Everson (LADR-A2ALL)[27]	44	59%	25%
GT 1/4/6	23	52%	22%
GT 2/3	21	67%	29%
Totals	192	40%	24%

Abbreviations: LADR-A2ALL, low accelerated dose regimen of PEG interferon/ribavirin, was conducted as a substudy of the NIH-sponsored Adult-to-Adult Living Donor Liver Transplantation (A2ALL) Study. Patients infected with genotypes (GT) 1, 4, 5, and 6 were randomized 2:1; treatment: control, and patients infected with genotypes 2 or 3 were treated. pTVR, posttransplant virologic response, is defined by undetectable HCV RNA at 12 weeks after transplantation (LTx).

Overall, 59 were treated and 20 were not. Doses of PEG interferon alpha-2b, starting at 0.75 µg/kg wk, and ribavirin (RBV), starting at 600 mg/d, were escalated as tolerated. Patients assigned to treatment versus control had similar baseline characteristics. Per protocol, 13 patients (22%) assigned to treatment and 0 patients (0%) assigned to control achieved viral clearance ($P = .03$). Among treated GT 1/4/6 patients, 23 of 30 received a transplant, of whom 22% achieved pTVR; among treated GT 2/3 patients 21/29 received a transplant, of whom 29% achieved pTVR (see **Table 1**). The likelihood of achieving pTVR was related to treatment duration—pTVR was 0%, 18%, and 50% in patients treated for less than 8, 8 to 16, and more than 16 weeks, respectively ($P = .01$) (**Fig. 1**). Treated patients experienced more serious adverse events (2.7/patient vs 1.3/patient, $P = .003$), particularly infection. These results indicated that pretransplant treatment with PEG/RBV could prevent posttransplant recurrence of HCV in selected patients. However, optimal results require 16 weeks or more of treatment and treatment is associated with increased risk of potentially serious complications.

Given the limitations of PEG/RBV and TT in patients with advanced liver disease or those on the transplant waiting list, most clinicians accept HCV reinfection of the allograft and wait to treat HCV after liver transplantation. Future therapy using interferon-free regimens of potent direct-acting antivirals will undoubtedly improve tolerability, reduce adverse events, enhance viral response, and magnify interest in pretransplant treatment. **Table 2** provides a framework for speculation regarding the potential role of pretransplant therapy using the emerging antiviral drugs.

STRATEGY 2: POSTTRANSPLANT TREATMENT

The goal of posttransplant antiviral treatment is to clear HCV infection (SVR, undetectable HCV RNA 12 weeks or more after treatment). Posttransplant patients may not tolerate interferon-based treatment and are prone to cytopenias, particularly anemia, and serious complications including infection, hepatic failure, and even death. Drug-drug interactions of immunosuppressants with either telaprevir or boceprevir complicate management.

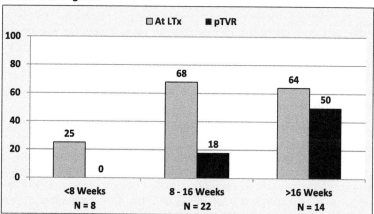

Pre-transplant Treatment: LADR-A2ALL

Fig. 1. Pretransplant treatment: Low accelerated dose regimen–Adult-to-Adult Living Donor Liver Transplantation Cohort Study. (*Data from* Everson GT, Terrault NA, Lok AS, et al. A2ALL Study. A randomized controlled trial of pretransplant antiviral therapy to prevent recurrence of hepatitis C after liver transplantation. Hepatology 2012.)

Table 2
Speculations regarding future drug regimens for pretransplant treatment, timelines, and outcomes

Genotype	Year	Treatment Options	Rate of SVR or pTVR	Optimum Duration of Treatment			Severity of Side Effects
				<8 wk	8–16 wk	>16 wk	
GT 2 or 3							
	2012	PR	29%–50%	-	-	100%	++++
	≥2013	R-NI	>65%	20%	80%	-	+
GT 1a or 1b							
	2012	PR	20%–25%	-	-	100%	
	2012	PR + PI-1st	40%	-	80%	20%	+++++
	≥2013	PR + PI-2nd	55%	-	80%	20%	+++
	≥2014	PR-5al	55%	-	80%	20%	+++
	≥2014	PR-NI	>60%	-	100%	-	++
	≥2014	R-NI	>55%	-	100%	-	+
	≥2014	Multi-DAA	>60%	20%	80%	-	++
GT 1b	≥2014	5al + PI-2nd	>60%	20%	80%	-	+
GT 1a	>2014	PR + 5al + PI-2nd	>60%	20%	80%	-	++

Abbreviations: 1st, first generation drug; 2nd, later generation drugs; 5al, inhibitor of NS5A protein; DAA, direct-acting antivirals; GT, genotype; NI, nucleos(t)ide-based inhibitor of NS5B polymerase; PI, inhibitor of NS3/4A protease; PR, peginterferon/ribavirin; pTVR, post-transplant virologic response (HCV RNA undetectable 12 weeks after transplantation); SVR, sustained virologic response; wk, weeks.

Prophylactic and preemptive antiviral strategies have not been proven effective. Most centers treat patients 6 months or more posttransplant who have active or aggressive HCV recurrence.[13,14,28]

Case 2: Treating a Patient After Liver Transplantation

A 61-year-old liver recipient with recurrent hepatitis C seeks treatment with TT 3 years after transplantation.

At year 1 posttransplant, the patient had active HCV, with grade 3 of 4 inflammation and stage 2 of 4 fibrosis. His immunosuppressive medications were tacrolimus 2 mg twice a day and mycophenolate mofetil 500 mg twice a day. He was treated with PEG/RBV for 48 weeks. HCV RNA was undetectable at week 24 of PEG/RBV and at end of treatment. He relapsed 4 weeks after treatment was discontinued. He describes the treatment as, "It nearly killed me!," and he experienced pancytopenia despite EPO and granulocyte colony-stimulating factor, mood changes, severe fatigue, and an overall poor sense of well-being.

Currently, the patient is asymptomatic with normal hemoglobin and WBC, bilirubin, INR, albumin, and creatinine. His ALT is 48 IU/mL, platelet count 99,000/μL, HCV RNA 10,000,000 IU/mL, HCV GT 1a, and IL28b genotype CT; liver biopsy now shows stage 3 fibrosis. His only immunosuppressive medication is sirolimus 2 mg every day. He has not experienced allograft rejection. Retreatment with TT using telaprevir is recommended.

Excluding poor tolerability to prior PEG/RBV, this case represents an excellent candidate for consideration of posttransplant treatment using TT. The characteristics that would favor successful treatment are as follows:

- Demonstrated sensitivity to interferon-based treatment
- Noncirrhotic stage of fibrosis

- Normal bilirubin, albumin, and INR
- No rejection

IL28b genotype CC also predicts the response to interferon-based treatment after liver transplantation. Both donor and recipient IL28b CC are associated with increased SVR in response to PEG/RBV; SVR is 90% in the cases where both donor and recipient are IL28b CC.[29]

PEG/RBV

Reviews of posttransplant antiviral therapy for HCV using PEG/RBV indicate SVRs of approximately 20% to –30% for GT 1 and approximately 60% to –70% for GT 2 or GT 3.[28–30] Approximately two-thirds of patients require dose reductions in PEG/RBV and approximately 25% discontinue treatment prematurely because of side effects or adverse events. Factors predicting SVR include naïve to posttransplant antiviral therapy, non-1 HCV genotype, RVR, relatively low HCV RNA at baseline, IL28b CC, low fibrosis stage, and adherence to treatment. Our patient had had a prior 48-week course of full-dose PEG/RBV and relapsed once treatment was discontinued. Because re-treatment with a second 48-week course of PEG/RBV would not likely clear his HCV infection, TT was recommended.

Case 2 (Continued)

Telaprevir and boceprevir are potent inhibitors of CYP3A, a key hepatic enzyme responsible for metabolism of many xenobiotics, including sirolimus, cyclosporine, and tacrolimus.[31–35] Doses of drugs metabolized by CYP3A must be reduced when using either telaprevir-based or boceprevir-based TT. Compared to sirolimus and tacrolimus, the pharmacokinetics of cyclosporine is least affected by telaprevir or boceprevir. The patient was treated under a protocol that entailed switching from sirolimus to cyclosporine/mycophenolate mofetil (MMF) (or mycophenolic acid [MFA]) and monitoring for rejection for 4 weeks, followed by a lead-in with PEG/RBV low accelerated dose regimen for 4 weeks, and then the addition of telaprevir. When telaprevir is added, cyclosporine dose is reduced.

TRIPLE THERAPY

Our protocols (University of Colorado) for treating HCV GT 1 in transplant recipients, using either telaprevir-based or boceprevir-based TT, are shown in **Figs. 2** and **3**. Remember, telaprevir-based and boceprevir-based TT have only been approved for HCV GT 1 infection. PEG/RBV is still the recommended treatment of non-1 genotypes. Both algorithms use the same basic principles—cyclosporine-based immunosuppression, lead-in with PEG/RBV low accelerated dose regimen, addition of telaprevir or boceprevir after lead-in, and modifications to treatment duration. Telaprevir is given for 12 weeks in all cases, and boceprevir is given for 32 weeks in those with eRVR, but for 44 weeks otherwise. The suppression of CYP3A by telaprevir or boceprevir reverses quickly once they are discontinued, so upward adjustment in immunosuppressive drugs and daily monitoring of drug levels are required to avoid precipitation of allograft rejection. Stop guidelines for both algorithms are similar to those recommended for the treatment of chronic hepatitis C in nontransplant patients.

Immunosuppression

The optimal immunosuppressive regimen for use during TT of posttransplant recurrent hepatitis C is not yet established. Our rationale for using cyclosporine-based immunosuppression over tacrolimus-based or sirolimus-based regimens was 2-fold. First,

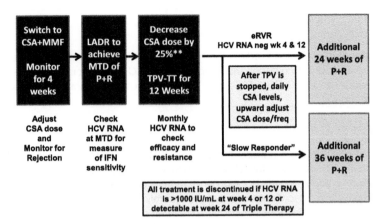

* TPV increases CSA exposure by 4- to 5-fold. If CSA total daily dose 200 mg, then change to 50 mg QD.

Fig. 2. Telaprevir use in the liver recipient. CSA, cyclosporine; MMF, mycophenolate mofetil; MTD, minimal tolerable dose; P+R, pegylated interferon + ribavirin; TPV-TT, telaprevir triple therapy.

cyclosporine may augment interferon-based antiviral therapy and enhance SVR. Cyclosporine is a weak antagonist of cyclophyllin-A, a host protein linked to HCV replication.[36] Also, in the ReViS-TC study, SVR was higher (48% vs 37%) and relapse was lower (18% vs 36%) when PEG/RBV treatment was used with cyclosporine-based versus tacrolimus-based immunosuppression.[37] Second, telaprevir or boceprevir impacts the pharmacokinetics of cyclosporine much less than tacrolimus, and presumably much less than either sirolimus or everolimus.[33,34] Because there is less deviation from standard monitoring procedures, presumably there is less risk for errors in the management of drug levels and dosage, and less risk for precipitating allograft rejection. **Table 3** shows the change in exposure to cyclosporine and tacrolimus when either telaprevir or boceprevir is used for antiviral treatment.

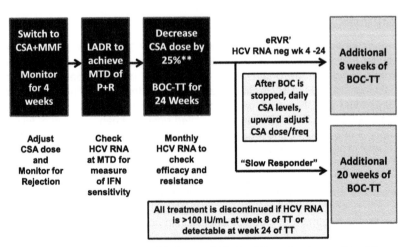

* BOC increases CSA exposure by 3-fold. If CSA total daily dose 200 mg, then change to 50 mg QD.

Fig. 3. Boceprevir use in the liver recipient. BOC_TT, boceprevir triple therapy; CSA, cyclosporine; MMF, mycophenolate mofetil; MTD, minimal tolerable dose; P+R, pegylated interferon + ribavirin.

Table 3		
Impact of boceprevir and telaprevir on pharmacokinetics of cyclosporine and tacrolimus[33,34]		
Increase in Single-dose CSA and TAC AUC due to multi-dose boceprevir or telaprevir (in healthy volunteers without chronic hepatitis C)		
	CSA	TAC[a]
Boceprevir	2.70	17.1
Telaprevir	4.64	70.3

Abbreviations: CSA, cyclosporin; TAC, tacrolimus.

[a] Sirolimus and Everolimus are expected to behave similarly to tacrolimus. No data available.

Data from Kiser JJ, Burton JR, Anderson PL, et al. Review and management of drug interactions with boceprevir and telaprevir. Hepatology 2012;55:1620–8.

PEG/RBV Lead-in

Although lead-in prolongs the overall treatment period, this strategy has important attributes. Switching immunosuppression may increase the risk for rejection and the subsequent addition of interferon may also increase risk for rejection. Lead-in provides a period for further monitoring to exclude precipitation of rejection. Also, the authors use an accelerating dose protocol so that during lead-in they define the maximum tolerated dose for PEG/RBV; this reduces fluctuations in PEG/RBV during subsequent TT. Maintaining stable PEG/RBV during telaprevir or boceprevir may reduce the risk for viral resistance and enhance SVR. The response in HCV RNA during lead-in is an indicator of sensitivity to interferon and may be a predictor of SVR. In nontransplant patients a greater than 1 $\log_{10}$ drop in HCV RNA during lead-in is an independent predictor of SVR[8,9]; our preliminary findings suggest that this is also true posttransplant.

Sequential Addition of Telaprevir or Boceprevir

The authors chose to add telaprevir or boceprevir to the antiviral regimen only after they had been assured that the patient was tolerating the switch in immunosuppression and had achieved maximal tolerated doses of PEG/RBV. With the addition of telaprevir or boceprevir, cyclosporine dose is reduced by 25%; for example, a patient taking 100 mg twice a day is reduced to 50 mg once a day. Levels of cyclosporine, both trough and C2, are closely monitored and doses are adjusted to maintain appropriate levels for maintenance of immunosuppression. The coadministration of MMF (or MFA) provides additional immunosuppression to prevent rejection. To date, using this protocol, no patient has experienced a rejection episode.

We have not observed any change in RBC, WBC, or platelet counts with the change to cyclosporine (CSA)/mycophenolate mofetil (MMF) immunosuppression but there is significant reduction in all 3 cell counts during PEG/RBV lead-in, and a major further decrease in RBC counts with addition of telaprevir.

Adjustment in Immunosuppressive Medication After Stopping Telaprevir or Boceprevir

The inhibition of CYP3A by telaprevir or boceprevir occurs immediately on administration of these drugs. Likewise, when telaprevir or boceprevir is discontinued, the inhibition of CYP3A ceases in accordance with the half-life of the disappearance of these compounds.[31–34] As a result, within 24 to 48 hours of the discontinuation of telaprevir and boceprevir, the activity of CYP3A is restored. Because these patients are on reduced doses of immunosuppression at the time telaprevir and boceprevir are discontinued, they are uniquely susceptible to allograft rejection because of the rapid reduction in immunosuppressive drug levels as CYP3A activity increases. For these reasons, it is imperative to monitor immunosuppressive blood levels closely and upward adjust doses of immunosuppressive therapy accordingly.

Case 2 (Continued)

Sirolimus was discontinued and cyclosporine 100 mg twice a day plus MMF 500 mg twice a day were initiated. After 4 weeks, PEG/RBV, 90 ug/wk/600 mg/d, was added and escalated to maximum tolerated doses of PEG 180 ug/wk and RBV 1000 mg/d. After an additional 4 weeks, telaprevir, 750 mg 3 times a day, was added, initiating TT, and cyclosporine was reduced to 50 mg every day. Trough and C2 levels of cyclosporine were measured twice weekly during the first 2 weeks.

HCV RNA was undetectable by week 4 of TT and the patient achieved eRVR. Telaprevir was discontinued after 12 weeks of TT, and PEG/RBV was continued for an additional 24 weeks. The patient had undetectable HCV RNA throughout, and HCV RNA remained undetectable 12 weeks posttreatment.

During therapy, the patient experienced the same side effects that he had during his first course of PEG/RBV, but the anemia was worse, requiring dose reductions in RBV, EPO, and blood transfusions.

ANTICIPATED OUTCOMES WITH TRIPLE THERAPY
Projected Rates of SVR

Assuming side effects and drug-drug interactions are managed appropriately, rates of SVR for HCV GT 1 should improve with TT. Nonetheless, posttransplant patients represent a group that is both "difficult to treat" and "difficult to cure." Recurrent hepatitis C in the liver recipient is characterized by high viral load and accelerated fibrosis, factors that impair response to interferon-based treatment. In addition, most of these patients have had prior courses of PEG/RBV either before or after liver transplantation and are relatively interferon resistant. An increasing stage of fibrosis and an impaired response to interferon impair the viral response to TT. Posttransplant immunosuppression may further impair the response to treatment.

Fig. 4A shows the impact on SVR of adding telaprevir or boceprevir to PEG/RBV in treatment-naïve, nontransplant patients (left bars). In the same figure, the right bars optimistically suggest that the posttransplant patient with HCV GT 1 should expect the same maximum improvement in SVR of approximately 30% and achieve a SVR of 60%. However, as demonstrated in **Fig. 4**B, and discussed earlier, the posttransplant patient has characteristics that impair viral responses, and perhaps a more realistic SVR in posttransplant patients is 45% to 50%. At the time of this writing, there were no reports of rates of SVR using TT in posttransplant patients.

On-treatment Viral Responses

Early reports from a few transplant centers have suggested that the use of TT posttransplant is associated with brisk early viral responses but that side effects and adverse events are common and may be serious, even life-threatening.

Mantry and colleagues[38] reported their experience in treating 7 patients with HCV GT 1 infection with telaprevir-based TT. Tacrolimus dose was reduced to a half-dose given weekly and blood concentrations were monitored closely. Six patients achieved undetectable HCV RNA by week 12, and 4 of these patients had undetectable HCV RNA at week 4 (eRVR). All of the patients had side effects; 6 patients had severe anemia requiring blood transfusions, and there was 1 death.

Kwo and colleagues[39] treated 7 patients with cirrhosis who were null responders to prior PEG/RBV treatment. All were converted to cyclosporine-based immunosuppression

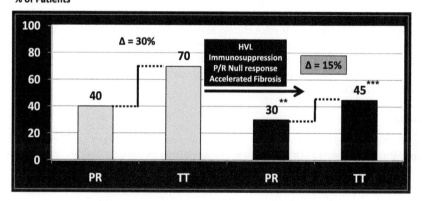

Fig. 4. The combined results from the ADVANCE and SPRINT-2 trials for both peginterferon/ribavirin (PR) and triple therapy (TT) are represented by the gray bars to the left in Panels A and B. Published results of PR therapy in liver recipients are represented by the black bar labeled PR to the right in Panels A and B. Estimated projections for SVR in transplant recipients treated with TT are represented by the black bars labeled TT to the right in Panels A and B. HVL, high viral load; PR or P/R, peginterferon/ribavirin; TT, triple therapy. (*Data from* Jacobson IM, McHutchison JG, Dusheiko G, et al. Telaprevir for previously untreated chronic hepatitis C virus infection. N Engl J Med 2011;364:2405–16; Poordad F, McCone J Jr, Bacon BR, et al. Boceprevir for untreated chronic HCV genotype 1 infection. N Engl J Med 2011;364:1195–206; Berenguer M. Systematic review of the treatment of established recurrent hepatitis C with pegylated interferon in combination with ribavirin. J Hepatology 2008;49:274–87; Wang CS, Ko HH, Yoshida EM, et al. Interferon-based combination anti-viral therapy for hepatitis C virus after liver transplantation: a review and quantitative analysis. Am J Transplant 2006;6(7):1586–99.)

before initiating TT. Five of the 7 patients achieved undetectable HCV RNA by week 12 of TT and HCV RNA remained undetectable at week 16. One of the 5 responders terminated TT early at week 10 because of hepatic decompensation. Anemia was severe. All patients required dose reduction in RBV and 6 of the 7 required EPO and blood transfusions. Five patients required granulocyte colony-stimulating factor for neutropenia, and 2 patients required eltrombopag for severe thrombocytopenia.

A French Multi-Center study reported results from 17 patients treated with boceprevir-based TT and 11 patients treated with telaprevir-based TT.[40] More than 50% of the patients were treatment-experienced and had advance fibrosis or cirrhosis. Immunosuppressive protocols were center-specific and varied. Rates of undetectable HCV RNA with boceprevir versus telaprevir were 35% versus 36% at week 4, and 56% versus 70% at week 8. Clinically significant anemia occurred in 71%, 90% received EPO, and 15% required blood transfusion.

Burton and Everson[41] used the treatment algorithm for telaprevir-based TT, as shown in **Fig. 2**, in 35 patients, 14 of whom had completed 12 weeks of TT. At week 1 after the addition of telaprevir, the mean HCV RNA had decreased by 6 $\log_{10}$; at week 4 of TT, 92% had HCV RNA <43 IU/mL (LOQ) and 50% had HCV RNA <18 IU/mL (LOD). Time to undetectable HCV RNA during TT predicted a breakthrough on PEG/RBV after stopping telaprevir—none of the patients clearing HCV RNA by week 6 experienced breakthrough; all slow responders (N = 3), who achieved undetectable HCV RNA after 6 weeks of TT, experienced breakthrough on PEG/RBV (**Fig. 5**). The decrease in HCV RNA during lead-in also predicted response during TT; 90% of patients with a more than 1 $\log_{10}$ drop in HCV RNA during lead-in had undetectable HCV RNA after 4 weeks of TT compared with 50% of patients with less than 1 $\log_{10}$ drop. Follow-up studies will determine the relationships of these early viral responses to SVR.

Anemia

Severe anemia has been the major management issue in treating patients after liver transplantation. Anemia during antiviral therapy is due to the combination of hemolysis from ribavirin and bone marrow suppression from interferon and telaprevir or boceprevir. Posttransplant patients may be further compromised by immunosuppressive

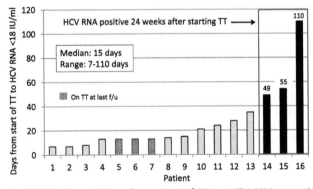

Fig. 5. Patients with the longest time from start of TT to HCV RNA negativity were ultimately HCV RNA positive at week 24. (*Courtesy of* James R. Burton Jr, MD.)

drugs. **Fig. 6** shows the sequential change in mean levels of hemoglobin in the Burton study using telaprevir-based TT. Hemoglobin did not change during the switch from tacrolimus or sirolimus to cyclosporine/MMF, but dropped by 1.5 g/dL during the lead-in with PEG/RBV, and dropped by another 2.5 g/dL in the first 1 to 4 weeks after the addition of telaprevir. Sixty-one percent (11/18) required EPO; 6 of the 11 who required EPO were started during PEG/RBV lead-in. Eighty-three percent (15/18) had RBV dose reduction after the addition of telaprevir. A majority (10/18) of patients required at least 1 blood transfusion with most (8/10) of these transfusions being given during the telaprevir phase of the protocol. Of the 10 patients receiving blood transfusion, a total of 60 units of blood was transfused, 48 units during the telaprevir phase of the protocol. This experience emphasizes that intervention for anemia is required early during TT; decreases in hemoglobin can be precipitous, and multiple approaches to control anemia may be needed simultaneously. The authors have since raised our hemoglobin threshold for RBV dose reduction and the addition of EPO from 10 g/dL to 11 g/dL.

Rash

Curiously, rash events have been extremely rare in transplant recipients. Rash has been reported in more than 50% of nontransplant patients taking telaprevir-based TT, and 5% to –7% of these patients have had to stop telaprevir because of severe rash. None of our posttransplant patients experienced rash. This observation suggests that the rash of telaprevir is dose-dependent or may have an immunologic basis that is blocked by the immunosuppressive therapies used in transplant recipients.

Drug-Drug Interactions

A major concern is the potential for toxicity from immunosuppressive drugs because of the blockade of their hepatic metabolism by telaprevir or boceprevir. Nearly all liver recipients take maintenance immunosuppression that is either tacrolimus-based, cyclosporine-based, or sirolimus-based. All 3 drugs are metabolized via the hepatic

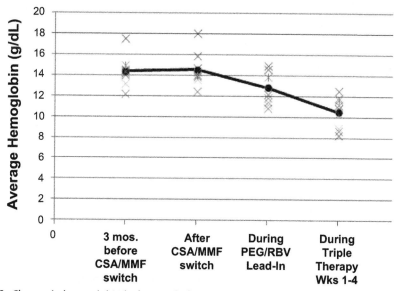

Fig. 6. Change in hemoglobin before and after triple therapy. CSA/MMF, cyclosporine/mycophenolate mofetil. (*Courtesy of* James R. Burton Jr, MD.)

enzyme CYP3A, an enzyme that is inhibited by both telaprevir and boceprevir. **Table 3** shows the relative increase in exposure from single doses of tacrolimus and cyclosporine in healthy volunteers taking telaprevir or boceprevir. The increase in exposure is most dramatic with tacrolimus, up to a 70-fold increase! Although only a 4-fold to 5-fold increase was observed with cyclosporine, this increase still represents a huge change from baseline immunosuppression. There are no studies with sirolimus or everolimus, but the impact is anticipated to be similar to that observed with tacrolimus. What this means to transplant hepatologists and patients is obvious: when using TT posttransplant, major reductions in doses of tacrolimus, cyclosporine, sirolimus, and everolimus are required and drug levels must be monitored closely.

The focus of drug-drug interactions has been on immunosuppressive drugs, because these effects are the most dramatic and have the greatest consequences. However, telaprevir and boceprevir may affect the metabolism of a wide array of medications, including antibiotics, sedatives, antipsychotics, statins, oral contraceptives, warfarin, proton-pump inhibitors, and others.[31,42] A careful consideration of all potential drug-drug interactions is required before initiating TT.

FUTURE DIRECTIONS FOR ANTIVIRAL HCV THERAPY

Several new drugs are currently in clinical trials for the treatment of chronic hepatitis C, including new types of interferons, second-generation and third-generation protease inhibitors, polymerase inhibitors, NS5A inhibitors, and others. Given the intolerance of pretransplant and posttransplant patients to interferon-based therapy, the rapidly evolving strategy of interferon-free treatment is particularly appealing.

Pegylated Interferon-Lambda

PEG interferon-lambda has demonstrated similar or enhanced viral responses compared with PEG interferon-alpha.[43] Its main advantages over standard PEG interferon-alpha include less bone marrow suppression with lower risk for anemia, neutropenia, and thrombocytopenia. This property of PEG interferon-lambda is advantageous when treating pretransplant and posttransplant patients. However, the other interferon side effects may limit its overall utility.

Immediately Emerging Direct-Acting Antivirals

Within 12 to 24 months, new direct-acting antivirals against HCV may become available.[44] The first in line seem to be the NS3/4A protease inhibitor, simeprevir, the NS5B polymerase inhibitor, sofusbivir, and the NS5A protein inhibitor, daclatasvir. All are in phase III trials for GT 1 infection in combination with PEG/RBV, and sofusbivir is in phase III trials for GT2/3 infection in combination with RBV (IFN-free regimen). Advantages of simeprevir over telaprevir or boceprevir include increased potency (potentially higher rates of SVR), daily dosing (as opposed to 3 times a day), and fewer, if any, side effects (no rash or anemia beyond that of the PEG/RBV backbone). The increased potency reduces but does not eliminate the risk for viral resistance.[45] Simeprevir undergoes hepatic metabolism and is prone to drug-drug interactions. Advantages of sofusbivir include high potency (SVR 91% with PEG/RBV in GT 1), high barrier to viral resistance,[45] daily dosing, lack of side effects, and renal clearance reducing risk for drug-drug interactions. Advantages of daclatasvir include high potency, daily dosing, and lack of side effects. Daclatasvir has a low barrier to viral resistance[45] and undergoes hepatic metabolism, making it prone to drug-drug interactions. Perhaps the most exciting aspect of these emerging drugs is that each targets a unique nonoverlapping component of the

HCV replication cycle. If one includes PEG and RBV, the palette of available therapies for treating HCV could soon encompass 5 classes of drug therapy!

Many drugs and drug combinations are entering late phase II or phase III testing, discussed in other articles in this series, and trials may be listed at www. clinicaltrials.gov, public web sites, or company web sites.

Interferon-free Treatment

Drawbacks of interferon, which are particularly problematic in pretransplant and post-transplant treatment, include low potency, a plethora of side effects, and the need for prolonged treatment (48 weeks or more in GT 1). However, most hepatologists who have treated hepatitis C over the last 2 decades have depended on interferon as the backbone for treatment. As recent as 2 years ago at a gathering of about 30 hepatologists, the question was posed, "Will interferon-free therapy be sufficient for success in treating HCV?" Most opined that only a minority of patients could be cured, and that interferon would remain a necessary component of the regimen. Only one suggested that interferon-free treatment could be successful in 100% of cases. Early reports seem to vindicate the enthusiasm of our optimistic colleague—interferon-free regimens are demonstrating rates of SVR exceeding 90%!

As drugs and treatment evolve, impressive results are currently being witnessed with interferon-free regimens in treating chronic hepatitis C.[46–53] Several new regimens are at the early stages of clinical development but could translate into major advances in both pretransplant and posttransplant treatment:

- Sofusbivir/RBV in HCV GT 2/3
- Sofusbivir/Daclatasvir ± RBV in HCV GT 1
- Sofusbivir/Simeprevir ± RBV in HCV GT 1

Table 4
Speculations regarding future drug regimens for post-transplant treatment, timelines, and outcomes

| Genotype | Year | Treatment Options | Rate of SVR | Optimum Duration of Treatment | | | Severity of Side Effects |
				12 wk	24 wk	48 wk	
GT 2 or 3							
	2012	PR	60%	-	50%	50%	+++
	≥2013	R-NI	>70%	50%	50%	-	+
GT 1a or 1b							
	2012	PR	30%	-	-	100%	
	2012	PR + PI-1st	45%	-	50%	50%	+++++
	≥2013	PR + PI-2nd	55%	-	80%	20%	+++
	≥2014	PR-5al	55%	-	80%	20%	+++
	≥2014	PR-NI	>60%	50%	50%	-	++
	≥2014	R-NI	>60%	-	100%	-	+
	≥2014	Multi-DAA	>60%	50%	50%	-	++
GT 1b	≥2014	5al + PI-2nd	>60%	-	100%	-	+
GT 1a	>2014	PR + 5al + PI-2nd	>60%	-	100%	-	++

Abbreviations: 1st, first generation drug; 2nd, later generation drugs; 5al, inhibitor of NS5A protein; DAA, direct-acting antivirals; GT, genotype; NI, nucleos(t)ide-based inhibitor of NS5B polymerase; PI, inhibitor of NS3/4A protease; PR, peginterferon/ribavirin; pTVR, post-transplant virologic response (HCV RNA undetectable 12 weeks after transplantation); SVR, sustained virologic response; wk, weeks.

- Sofusbivir/GS-5885 ± RBV in HCV GT 1
- Daclatasvir/Simeprevir ± RBV in HCV GT 1
- Daclatasvir/Asunaprevir in HCV GT 1b
- Daclatasvir/Asunaprevir/non-Nuc NS5B inhibitor in HCV GT 1
- ABT-450/r/ABT-267/ABT-333(or -072) + RBV in HCV GT 1
- Other combinations

As the palette of therapeutic options expands, it is highly likely that nearly all of the patients undergoing liver transplantation for chronic hepatitis C could be successfully treated before or after transplantation! **Table 4** provides speculations on regimens, timelines, treatment durations, and potential outcomes.

SUMMARY

Telaprevir and boceprevir have ushered in a new era of direct-acting antiviral therapy in the treatment of HCV infection. Rapid advances in new drug therapy promise to improve overall outcomes, reduce side effects, shorten treatment duration, simplify treatment regimens, and lower the risk for drug-drug interactions. Ultimately, interferon-free therapy may emerge as the treatment standard. How should the transplant hepatologist react to these rapidly changing paradigms? The authors personally believe that it is their prerogative to encourage, if not demand, targeted clinical trials of new drug therapy for both pretransplant and posttransplant patients. Until other options come available, treatment choices are limited to either PEG/RBV (all GTs) or TT (only GT 1). The emerging data suggest that current TT should be used with caution by experienced clinicians in liver centers and with very close monitoring of side effects and adverse events. Drug-drug interactions are common and potentially dangerous. The transplant hepatologist must be prepared to lower immunosuppression and closely monitor drug levels at the onset of TT, increase immunosuppression, and closely monitor drug levels when telaprevir or boceprevir are stopped. The hope of future treatments includes pangenotype coverage, reduced side effects, lack of bone marrow suppression, elimination of drug-drug interactions, and ultimately Food and Drug Administration–approved indications for use of antiviral treatment before and after liver transplantation. Patients will benefit, but the question is when? Transplant hepatologists, pharmaceutical partners, and liver recipients should work together to push up the timelines!

REFERENCES

1. Wiesner RH, Sorrell M, Villamil F. Report of the first International Liver Transplantation Society expert panel consensus conference on liver transplantation and hepatitis C. Liver Transpl 2003;9:S1–9.
2. Ghany MG, Nelson DR, Strader DB, et al, American Association for Study of Liver Diseases. An update on treatment of genotype 1 chronic hepatitis C virus infection: 2011 practice guideline by the American Association for the Study of Liver Diseases. Hepatology 2011;54:1433–44.
3. Selzner N, Renner EL, Selzner M, et al. Antiviral treatment of recurrent hepatitis C after liver transplantation: predictors of response and long-term outcome. Transplantation 2009;88:1214–21.
4. Kornberg A, Küpper B, Tannapfel A, et al. Sustained clearance of serum hepatitis C virus-RNA independently predicts long-term survival in liver transplant patients with recurrent hepatitis C. Transplantation 2008;86(3):469–73.

5. Jacobson IM, McHutchison JG, Dusheiko G, et al. Telaprevir for previously untreated chronic hepatitis C virus infection. N Engl J Med 2011;364:2405–16.
6. Sherman KE, Flamm SL, Afdhal NH, et al. Response-guided telaprevir combination treatment for hepatitis C virus infection. N Engl J Med 2011;365:1014–24.
7. Zeuzem S, Andreone P, Pol S, et al. Telaprevir for retreatment of HCV infection. N Engl J Med 2011;364:2417–28.
8. Poordad F, McCone J Jr, Bacon BR, et al. Boceprevir for untreated chronic HCV genotype 1 infection. N Engl J Med 2011;364:1195–206.
9. Bacon BR, Gordon SC, Lawitz E, et al. Boceprevir for previously treated chronic HCV genotype 1 infection. N Engl J Med 2011;364:1207–17.
10. Fried MW, Shiffman ML, Reddy KR, et al. Peginterferon alfa-2a plus ribavirin for chronic hepatitis C virus infection. N Engl J Med 2002;347:975–82.
11. Hadziyannis SJ, Sette H Jr, Morgan TR, et al. Peginterferon-alpha2a and ribavirin combination therapy in chronic hepatitis C: a randomized study of treatment duration and ribavirin dose. Ann Intern Med 2004;140:346–55.
12. Manns MP, McHutchison JG, Gordon SC, et al. Peginterferon alfa-2b plus ribavirin compared with interferon alfa-2b plus ribavirin for initial treatment of chronic hepatitis C: a randomised trial. Lancet 2001;358:958–65.
13. Roche B, Samuel D. Hepatitis C virus treatment pre- and post- liver transplantation. Liver Int 2012;32:120–8.
14. Saxena V, Terrault N. Hepatitis C virus treatment and liver transplantation in the era of new antiviral therapies. Curr Opin Organ Transplant 2012;17:216–24.
15. Ge D, Fellay J, Thompson AJ, et al. Genetic variation in IL28B predicts hepatitis C treatment-induced viral clearance. Nature 2009;461:399–401.
16. Clark PJ, Thompson AJ. Host genomics and HCV treatment response. J Gastroenterol Hepatol 2012;27(2):212–22.
17. Hezode C, Dorival C, Zoulim F, et al. Real-life safety of telaprevir or boceprevir in combination with peginterferon alfa/ribavirin in cirrhotic nonresponders: First results of the French early access program (ANRS CO20-CUPIC). Presented at HEPDART December 4–8, 2011, Kauai, HI, USA. Global Antiviral Journal 2011;7:54A.
18. Iacobellis A, Siciliano M, Perri F, et al. Peginterferon alfa-2b and ribavirin in patients with hepatitis C virus and decompensated cirrhosis: a controlled study. J Hepatol 2007;46:206–12.
19. Amarapurkar DN, Patel ND, Kamani P. Antiviral therapy of decompensated cirrhosis due to hepatitis C viral infection. Trop Gastroenterol 2005;26:119–22.
20. Annicchiarico BE, Siciliano M, Avolio AW, et al. Treatment of chronic hepatitis C virus infection with pegylated interferon and ribavirin in cirrhotic patients awaiting liver transplantation. Transplant Proc 2008;40:1918–20.
21. Carrion JA, Martinez-Bauer E, Crespo G, et al. Antiviral therapy increases the risk of bacterial infections in HCV-infected cirrhotic patients awaiting liver transplantation: a retrospective study. J Hepatol 2009;50:719–28.
22. Crippin JS, McCashland T, Terrault N, et al. A pilot study of the tolerability and efficacy of antiviral therapy in hepatitis C virus-infected patients awaiting liver transplantation. Liver Transpl 2002;8:350–5.
23. Forns X, Garcia-Retortillo M, Serrano T, et al. Antiviral therapy of patients with decompensated cirrhosis to prevent recurrence of hepatitis C after liver transplantation. J Hepatol 2003;39:389–96.
24. Tekin F, Gunsar F, Karasu Z, et al. Safety, tolerability, and efficacy of pegylated-interferon alfa-2a plus ribavirin in HCV-related decompensated cirrhotics. Aliment Pharmacol Ther 2008;27:1081–5.

25. Thomas RM, Brems JJ, Guzman-Hartman G, et al. Infection with chronic hepatitis C virus and liver transplantation: a role for interferon therapy before transplantation. Liver Transpl 2003;9:905–15.

26. Everson GT, Trotter J, Forman L, et al. Treatment of advanced hepatitis C with a low accelerating dosage regimen of antiviral therapy. Hepatology 2005;42:255–62.

27. Everson GT, Terrault NA, Lok AS, et al, A2ALL Study. A randomized controlled trial of pretransplant antiviral therapy to prevent recurrence of hepatitis c after liver transplantation. Hepatology 2012. [Epub ahead of print]. http://dx.doi.org/10.1002/hep.25976.

28. Berenguer M. Systematic review of the treatment of established recurrent hepatitis C with pegylated interferon in combination with ribavirin. J Hepatology 2008; 49:274–87.

29. Duarte-Rojo A, Veldt BJ, Goldstein DD, et al. The course of posttransplant hepatitis c infection: comparative impact of donor and recipient source of the favorable IL28B genotype and other variables. Transplantation 2012;94(2): 197–203.

30. Wang CS, Ko HH, Yoshida EM, et al. Interferon-based combination anti-viral therapy for hepatitis C virus after liver transplantation: a review and quantitative analysis. Am J Transplant 2006;6(7):1586–99.

31. Kiser JJ, Burton JR, Anderson PL, et al. Review and management of drug interactions with boceprevir and telaprevir. Hepatology 2012;55:1620–8.

32. Garg V, Kauffman RS, Beaumont M, et al. Telaprevir: pharmacokinetics and drug interactions. Antivir Ther 2012. [Epub ahead of print]. http://dx.doi.org/10.3851/IMP2356.

33. Garg V, van Heeswijk R, Lee JE, et al. Effect of telaprevir on the pharmacokinetics of cyclosporine and tacrolimus. Hepatology 2011;54(1):20–7. http://dx.doi.org/10.1002/hep.24443.

34. Hulskotte E, Gupta S, Xuan F, et al. Pharmacokinetic interaction between the HCV protease inhibitor boceprevir and cyclosporine and tacrolimus in healthy volunteers. Hepatology 2012. [Epub ahead of print]. http://dx.doi.org/10.1002/hep.25831.

35. Rabie R, Mumtaz K, Renner EL. Efficacy of antiviral therapy for hepatitis C post liver transplant on cyclosporine versus tacrolimus: a systematic review and meta-analysis. Liver Transpl 2012. [Epub ahead of print]. http://dx.doi.org/10.1002/lt.23516.

36. Nag A, Robotham JM, Tang H. Suppression of viral RNA binding and the assembly of infectious hepatitis C virus particles in vitro by cyclophilin inhibitors. J Virol 2012. [Epub ahead of print].

37. ReViS-TC Study Group. Cyclosporine a-based immunosuppression reduces relapse rate after antiviral therapy in transplanted patients with hepatitis C virus infection: a large multicenter cohort study. Transplantation 2011;92(3):334–40.

38. Mantry PS, Hassett MS, Weinstein J, et al. Triple therapy using telaprevir in the treatment of hepatitis C recurrence after liver transplantation: an early single center experience (Liver Institute at Methodist Dallas Medical Center, Dallas, TX, USA). Presented at HEPDART, December 4–8, 2011, Kauai, Hawaii. Global Antiviral Journal 2011;7:87A.

39. Kwo PY, Ghabril M, Lacerda MA, et al. 845 use of telaprevir plus PEG interferon/ribavirin for null responders post OLT with advanced fibrosis/cholestatic hepatitis C. Gastroenterology 2012;142:S934.

40. Coilly A, Roche B, Botta-Fridlund D, et al. A first multicentric experience of protease inhibitors for severe hepatitis C recurrence after liver transplantation. Liver Transpl 2012;18:S84.

41. Burton JR, Everson GT. Initial experience with telaprevir for treating hepatitis C virus in liver recipients: virologic response, safety, and tolerability. Am J Transplant 2012;LB1 (Presented at ATC, 2012).
42. Wilby KJ, Greanya ED, Ford JAE, et al. A review of drug interactions with boceprevir and telaprevir: implications for HIV and transplant patients. Ann Hepatol 2012;11:179–82.
43. Muir AJ, Shiffman ML, Zaman A, et al. Phase 1b study of pegylated interferon lambda 1 with or without ribavirin in patients with chronic genotype 1 hepatitis C virus infection. Hepatology 2010;52:822–32.
44. Pockros PJ. Drugs in development for chronic hepatitis C: a promising future. Expert Opin Biol Ther 2011;11:1611–22.
45. Pawlotsky JM. Treatment failure and resistance with direct-acting antiviral drugs against hepatitis C virus. Hepatology 2011;53:1742–51.
46. Lawitz E, Poordad F, Kowdley KV, et al. A 12-week interferon-free regimen of ABT-450/r, ABT-072, and ribavirin was well tolerated and achieved sustained virologic response in 91% of treatment-naïve HCV IL28B-CC genotype-1-infected subjects. J Hepatology 2012;56:S7.
47. Gane EJ, Roberts SK, Stedman CA, et al. Oral combination therapy with a nucleoside polymerase inhibitor (RG7128) and danoprevir for chronic hepatitis C genotype 1 infection (INFORM-1): a randomised, double-blind, placebo-controlled, dose-escalation trial. Lancet 2010;376:1467–75.
48. Lok AS, Gardiner DF, Lawitz E, et al. Preliminary study of two antiviral agents for hepatitis C genotype 1. N Engl J Med 2012;366:216–24.
49. Suzuki F, Ikeda K, Toyota J, et al. Dual oral therapy with the NS5A inhibitor daclatasvir (BMS-790052) and NS3 protease inhibitor Asunaprevir (BMS-650032) in HCV genotype 1B-Infected null responders or Ineligible/Intolerant to Peginterferon/Ribavirin. J Hepatology 2012;56:S7.
50. Chayama K, Takahashi S, Toyota J, et al. Dual therapy with the NS5A inhibitor BMS-790052 and the NS3 protease inhibitor BMS-650032 in HCV genotype 1b-infected null responders. Hepatology 2012;55:742–8.
51. Zeuzem S, Sorano V, Asselah T, et al. SVR4 and SVR12 with an interferon-free regimen of BI201335 and BI207127, ± ribavirin, in treatment-naïve patients with chronic genotype-1 HCV infection: interim results of SOUND-C2. J Hepatology 2012;56:S45.
52. Poordad F, Lawitz E, Kowdley KV, et al. 12-Week interferon-free regimen of ABT-450/r + ABT-333 + ribavirin achieved SVR12 in more than 90% of treatment-naïve genotype-1-infected subjects and 47% of previous non-responders. J Hepatology 2012;56:S549.
53. Sulkowski M, Rodriguez-Torres M, Lawitz E, et al. High sustained virologic response rate in treatment-naïve HCV genotype 1A and 1B patients treated for 12 weeks with an interferon-free all-oral QUAD regimen: interim results. J Hepatology 2012;56:S560.

Update on Combinations of DAAs With and Without Pegylated-Interferon and Ribavirin

Triple and Quadruple Therapy More Than Doubles SVR

Valérie Martel-Laferrière, MD*, Douglas T. Dieterich, MD

KEYWORDS

- Hepatitis C • Combination therapy • Monotherapy • Pegylated-interferon free

KEY POINTS

- Monotherapy is an ineffective strategy for the treatment of hepatitis C.
- The use of quadruple therapy combining pegylated-interferon, ribavirin, and 2 new direct-acting agents can lead to almost 100% sustained virologic response rates.
- Pegylated-inteferon free combinations are promising in early trials, but are not yet optimized.

INTRODUCTION

Standard interferon (IFN) has been approved for the treatment of hepatitis C (HCV) since 1991. Ribavirin (RBV), the last new drug for HCV until 2011, was approved in 1998 and pegylated-interferon (pegIFN) in 2002. Nine years passed before the approval of boceprevir (BOC) and telaprevir (TVR). In the next 10 years, the number of new drugs approved will multiply exponentially. When only 2 drugs were available, the question to combine them or not was irrelevant, but with drugs of different classes,

Funding sources: Valérie Martel-Laferrière: 2011 AMMI Canada/Pfizer Post Residency Fellowship; Douglas T. Dieterich: None.

Conflict of interest: Valérie Martel-Laferrière: None; Douglas T. Dieterich serves as a paid lecturer, consultant, and serves on scientific advisory boards of companies that either develop or assess medicines used for the treatment of viral hepatitis. These companies include Gilead Sciences, Boehringer Ingelheim, Novartis, Biolex, Pharmasset, Inhibitex, Vertex Pharmaceuticals, Achillion, Tibotec, Idenix, Pfizer, Merck, Kadmon, Bayer Healthcare, Genentech, Hoffman-La Roche Inc, and Bristol-Myers Squibb.

Division of Liver Diseases, Department of Medicine, Mount Sinai School of Medicine, One Gustave L. Levy Place, New York, NY 10029, USA

* Corresponding author.

E-mail address: valerie.martel-laferriere@mountsinai.org

Clin Liver Dis 17 (2013) 93–103

http://dx.doi.org/10.1016/j.cld.2012.09.001

potency, and resistance profiles, it will become essential to determine how drugs can be combined to optimize sustained virologic response (SVR) while reducing resistance and side effects.

Most of the agents currently being developed for the treatment of HCV are initially tested with pegIFN and RBV. The outcomes of these trials may be revised in other reviews. Now that more and more agents are being developed, pharmaceutical companies have begun to combine them in triple-therapy and quadruple-therapy regimens, both intercompany and intracompany. There are 2 main goals to combination therapy: improving SVR rates and avoiding the use of pegIFN. Currently, with the exception of 1 trial, the quadruple therapy combinations have been designed to optimize SVR rates and have retained pegIFN. Triple and quadruple combination therapies without pegIFN represent a ground-breaking advancement in HCV treatment. The purpose of this review was to explain the rationale of combination therapy and the triple and quadruple combination trials for which preliminary results are available.

COMBINATION THERAPY TO INCREASE ANTIVIRAL POTENCY

Over time, monotherapy has been tried for different drugs with more or less success. Standard IFN monotherapy was the first HCV treatment, even before the discovery of the virus. With IFN monotherapy, the SVR rates were approximately 15% to 20%. The combination of RBV added to IFN and, later, to pegIFN, increased the SVR rates to approximately 40% to 60% for genotype 1 and 4 and 70% to 80% for genotypes 2 and 3. This demonstrated for the first time that combination therapy was more potent than monotherapy for the treatment of HCV. Since the addition of RBV, IFN monotherapy is not a treatment option anymore, except in very specific situations, such as with patients on dialysis. RBV monotherapy has been evaluated in a Cochrane metanalysis.[1] In 14 randomized controlled trials including 657 patients, RBV monotherapy did not increase SVR rates when compared with placebo. It also did not affect liver morbidity or all-cause mortality.

Monotherapy with direct-acting antiviral agents (DAAs) is tested with most of the new agents during the first phases of clinical trials. Some have been tested in monotherapy in more advanced phases of research. As an example, TVR monotherapy was compared with a combination of TVR and pegIFN for 14 days.[2] The addition of pegIFN to the regimen changed the virologic decline from −3.99 log to −5.49 log. Four of the 8 patients on TVR/pegIFN were undetectable after 2 weeks versus 1 of the 8 patients on TVR monotherapy. Even one of the most potent drugs in trials, the nucleotide NS5B polymerase inhibitor GS-7977, was unable to prove its usefulness in monotherapy.[3] In the only monotherapy arm of the ELECTRON trial, only 60% of HCV genotype 2 or 3 treatment-naïve patients achieved SVR24 after a 12-week treatment versus 100% for those who received GS-7977 with RBV. All the patients who failed were undetectable at the end of the treatment but rapidly relapsed. No mutations were identified and resistance could not therefore explain the relapses. A potency problem is probably more the cause. The question remains whether the treatment was not long enough or was unable to reach all the HCV sanctuaries.

COMBINATION THERAPY TO DECREASE VIRAL RESISTANCE

HCV has a rapid replication rate with approximately 10^{12} virions produced per day.[4] Its RNA polymerase does not have proofreading ability.[4] This leads to the generation of multiple quasispecies, including some with potential for resistance to treatment. Rong and colleagues[4] estimated, based on the replication and replication error rates, that all possible single and double mutants are produced multiple times every day. Hopefully, not all of these mutants would be fit or viable. Rong and colleagues[4] also estimated that even with a very potent agent able to induce a viral decline of 5 log in 1 day, the number of viruses produced that day would be sufficient to generate all the single mutants.[4] The double and triple mutants would then be generated by additional mutations. This analysis theoretically showed that resistance mutations are inevitable during treatment. The goal is to find a way to overcome them.

Combination therapy allows a more rapid virologic decline. Fewer resistant variants should be generated. As the different agents usually act on different targets and are not affected by the same mutations, combination therapy may overcome DAA resistance.

QUADRUPLE THERAPY WITH PEGYLATED-INTERFERON

The Boehringer Ingelheim SOUND-C1 trial is a phase Ib study designed for treatment-naïve patients with genotype 1 who are not cirrhotic (**Box 1, Fig. 1A, Table 1**).[5] BI201335, a protease inhibitor, and BI207127, a non-nucleoside NS5B polymerase inhibitor, were combined with pegIFN and RBV. It is a sequential quadruple therapy trial. For the first 4 weeks, patients were exposed to B20135 120 mg every day, BI207127 (400 mg 3 times a day for arm A and 600 mg 3 times a day for arm B), and RBV. From week 5 to week 24, patients were treated with BI201335, pegIFN alfa 2a, and RBV. At week 24, patients who had a viral load of 25 IU/mL or less at week 4 and were undetectable at weeks 5 and 18 were stopped, whereas the others continued pegIFN and RBV until week 48. SVR was achieved by 73% and 94% of patients in arms A and B respectively. Twenty-four weeks of treatment was possible for 27% and 71% of the patients respectively. During the pegIFN-free 4-week treatment, 1 patient had a relapse and 1 had a 0.7 log rebound. The 2 patients continued the study. The first was undetectable when lost to follow-up and the second achieved SVR. The 2 patients had an R155K mutation in NS3 and the first patient also had a P495L in the NS5B. There was no virologic breakthrough during the rest of the treatment but there were 2 relapses.

ZENITH is a Vertex trial for genotype 1 treatment-naïve patients.[6] It combines VX-222, a non-nucleoside NS5B polymerase inhibitor, with TVR 1125 mg twice a day, pegIFN, and RBV. The study uses a response-guided therapy (RGT) approach

---

Box 1
Take-home messages from pegIFN quadruple therapy trials

Overall

- Quadruple therapy can achieve almost 100% SVR rate.

SOUND-C1

- Dual therapy leads to viral breakthrough that was overcome by addition of pegIFN and RBV.

ZENITH

- Quadruple therapy may overcome the impact of IL28B.

- SVR not available for the last 2 arms, but if favorable results, can be a way to safely avoid pegIFN in some patients.

Gilead

- Initial combination therapy has an impact on viral decrease and RVR rates.

AI447-011

- Quadruple therapy in null responders can lead to almost 100% SVR rates.

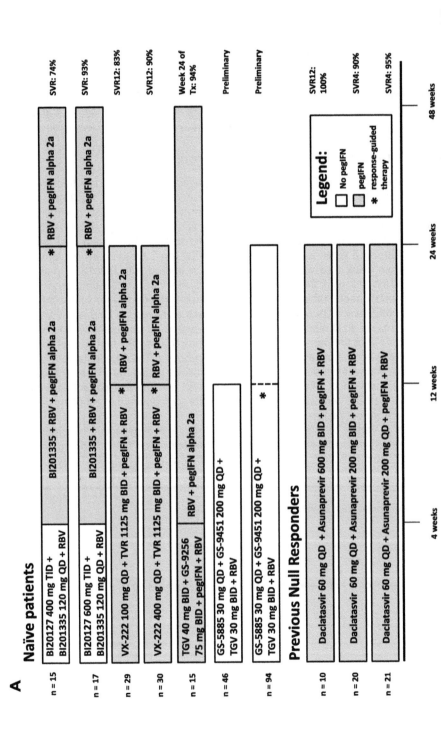

Fig. 1. (A) Design and outcomes of selected quadruple therapy arms. (B) Design and outcomes of selected triple-therapy arms. BID, 2 times daily; QD, once a day; TGV, tegobuvir; TID, 3 times daily.

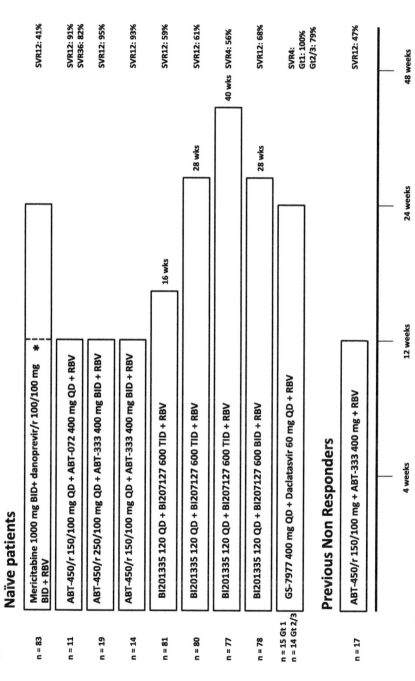

B

Naïve patients

n = 83 — Mercitabine 1000 mg BID + danoprevir/r 100/100 mg BID + RBV   *   — SVR12: 41%

n = 11 — ABT-450/r 150/100 mg QD + ABT-072 400 mg QD + RBV — SVR12: 91% SVR36: 82%

n = 19 — ABT-450/r 250/100 mg QD + ABT-333 400 mg BID + RBV — SVR12: 95%

n = 14 — ABT-450/r 150/100 mg QD + ABT-333 400 mg BID + RBV — SVR12: 93%

n = 81 — BI201335 120 QD + BI207127 600 TID + RBV — 16 wks — SVR12: 59%

n = 80 — BI201335 120 QD + BI207127 600 TID + RBV — 28 wks — SVR12: 61%

n = 77 — BI201335 120 QD + BI207127 600 TID + RBV — 40 wks SVR4: 56%

n = 78 — BI201335 120 QD + BI207127 600 BID + RBV — 28 wks — SVR12: 68%

n = 15 Gt 1
n = 14 Gt 2/3 — GS-7977 400 mg QD + Daclatasvir 60 mg QD + RBV — SVR4: Gt1: 100% Gt2/3: 79%

Previous Non Responders

n = 17 — ABT-450/r 150/100 mg + ABT-333 400 mg + RBV — SVR12: 47%

4 weeks   12 weeks   24 weeks   48 weeks

Fig. 1. (continued)

Table 1
Quadruple and triple combinations

	Protease Inhibitor	NS5A Polymerase Inhibitor	Non-Nucleoside NS5B Polymerase Inhibitor	Nucleos(t)ide NS5B Polymerase Inhibitor	Ribavirin	Pegylated-interferon
SOUND-C1	BI201335		BI207127		+	+
Zenith	Telaprevir		VX-222		±	±
Gilead	GS-9256		Tegobuvir		+	+
AI447-011	Asunaprevir	Daclatasvir			±	±
AI447-011 Expansion Cohort	Asunaprevir	Daclatasvir			+	+
INFORM-SVR	Danoprevir/r			Mericitabine	+	−
PILOT (M12-267)	ABT-450/r		ABT-072		+	−
CO-PILOT (M12-746)	ABT-450/r		ABT-333		+	−
SOUND-C2	BI201335		BI207127		±	−
AI444-040		Daclatasvir		GS-7977	±	−
Gilead all-oral quad (NCT01353248)	GS-9451	GS-5885	Tegobuvir		+	−

Abbreviations: +, in all arms; ±, in some arms; −, not included in the study.

with discontinuation at week 12 of treatment if patients are undetectable at weeks 2 and 8. Initially, arms A and B were 12 weeks of VX222 (100 mg every day or 400 mg every day) and TVR followed by pegIFN and RBV for 24 weeks if the patients did not meet the criteria for a 12-week treatment. Because of viral breakthrough in more than 25% of the patients, these arms were discontinued. The arms C and D combine VX-222 (100 mg every day versus 400 mg every day) with TVR, pegIFN, and RBV for the first 12 weeks and the patients who are not eligible for RGT continue treatment for another 12 weeks with pegIFN and RBV only. Arm E is exclusively for genotype 1b, whereas arm F is for genotype 1a. Patients are potentially pegIFN free as they combine VX-222 400 mg every day, TVR, and RBV for the first 12 weeks and pegIFN and RBV are continued for 24 weeks only if needed. SVR12 data are available for the arms C and D with 83% and 90% respectively (including 2 patients in arm C and 1 in arm D for which posttreatment week 12 data are missing). There was a 7% relapse rate in both groups. For the patients who were eligible for a 12-week treatment, 82% and 93% achieved SVR 24. Those who did not meet the criteria for RGT had an SVR12 rate of 83% and 87%. Of interest, IL28B polymorphism did not affect the SVR.[7] Because treatment is longer in the arms E and F, the SVR 12 data for the entire cohort are not yet available. For the 11 patients who were eligible for RGT and who consequently had a pegIFN-free treatment, 9 achieved SVR4 (5/5 genotype 1b and 4/6 genotype 1a).[8]

The Gilead Sciences quadruple trial with pegIFN was designed for genotype 1 treatment-naïve patients who are not cirrhotic.[9] It includes tegobuvir (GS-9190), a nonnucleoside NS5B polymerase inhibitor; GS-9256, a protease inhibitor; pegIFN; and RBV. It includes 3 arms: tegobuvir and GS-9256 alone or with RBV or with pegIFN/RBV for 4 weeks followed by pegIFN and RBV for 44 weeks. Rapid virologic response (RVR) results of this study emphasize the impact on antiviral potency of combination therapy as 7% achieved RVR if on dual therapy versus 38% if on triple therapy and 100% on quadruple therapy. The patients on dual therapy had an initial decrease of the virus for the first 7 days but then rebounded. With RBV, there was a decrease for 14 days that was generally maintained. With pegIFN/RBV, the decrease continued for 28 days. SVR24 was achieved by 67%, 100%, and 94% of the patients if they were initially on dual, triple, or quadruple therapy respectively.

The AI447-011 study of Bristol-Meyers Squibb is an open-label phase IIa study that was presented at the International Conference of the European Association for Study of the Liver in 2011.[10] It was designed for genotype 1 previous null responders. It is the first study to demonstrate that SVR could be achieved without pegIFN. The combination of daclatasvir 60 mg every day, an NS5A inhibitor, and asunaprevir 600 mg twice a day, an NS3 protease inhibitor, for 24 weeks led to a 36% SVR12. But the quadruple-therapy arm (daclatasvir/asunaprevir/pegIFN/RBV for 24 weeks) of this study is almost as important as the pegIFN-free arm. All the 10 patients achieved SVR12, demonstrating that, even in the most difficult-to-treat populations, nearly all patients can be cured with combination therapy. As a comparison, 38% of null responders on BOC and 37% of those on TVR achieved SVR.[11,12] Of interest in this study, the investigators reported lower rates for SVR24 and 48 but specify that the patient who relapsed had viral loads lower than the level of quantification and were undetectable again when retested a few days later. This supports the study of Harrington and colleagues[13] that showed that viral loads lower than the level of quantification should be considered during treatment with DAAs but usually represent false-positive results posttreatment. Other arms were later added to confirm the result of AI447-011 and to evaluate the dose of asunaprevir needed and the need for pegIFN and RBV.[14] Results are available for the 2 arms combining daclatasvir 60 mg every day, asunaprevir

200 mg (twice a day versus every day), pegIFN, and RBV for 24 weeks. SVR4 was achieved by 90% and 95% of the patients in the twice-a-day and every-day arms respectively. One patient in the twice-a-day arm relapsed, whereas the other patients who were detectable were lower than the level of quantification.

TRIPLE PEGIFN-FREE THERAPY

The INFORM-SVR study is a Roche phase IIb trial for genotype 1 treatment-naïve patients (**Box 2**, see **Fig. 1**B, **Table 1**).[15] It combines mericitabine, a nucleoside NS5B polymerase inhibitor; danoprevir, a protease inhibitor; ritonavir, a booster for danoprevir; and RBV or placebo. This study uses RGT where patients with a viral load of less than 43 IU/mL at weeks 2 and 8 and undectable at week 10 were re-randomized to stop treatment at week 12 or 24 (1:1), whereas the others continued until week 24. The 12-week arm with RBV and all the placebo arms were discontinued because of high relapse rates. Overall, 41% of patients achieved SVR 24 with an important difference between the patients who were genotype 1a (26%) versus 1b (71%). The patients eligible for an RGT but treated for 24 weeks had higher SVR rates (31% vs 17% for genotype 1a and 80% vs 64% for genotype 1b). The genotype seems to have a more important impact on treatment outcome than IL28B polymorphism. In the CC group, 32% of patients achieved SVR12 (27% for genotype 1a and 50% for genotype 1b). In the CT/TT group, it was 44% who achieved SVR12 (25% for genotype 1a and 76% for genotype 1b).

Abbott Laboratories presented 2 studies, PILOT (M12-267) and CO-PILOT (M12-746), at the European Association for the Study of the Liver meeting in 2012.[16,17] PILOT included 11 genotype 1 treatment-naïve patients with IL28B CC polymorphism and without cirrhosis or bridging fibrosis.[16] It is important to notice that this is a highly selected population and that results need to be considered as a proof of concept and are not reliable for the overall hepatitis C population. Eight patients with genotype 1a and 3 with genotype 1b were enrolled. The treatment combined ABT-450, an NS3 protease inhibitor used in combination with ritonavir, ABT-072, a non-nucleoside NS5B polymerase inhibitor, and RBV. All patients achieved RVR and were undetectable

---

Box 2
Take-home messages from pegIFN-free triple therapy trials

Overall
- Proof of concept: SVR is achievable without pegIFN.
- Oral combinations need optimization to improve the SVR rates.

INFORM-SVR
- Higher impact of the genotype (1a vs 1b) than the IL28B polymorphism.

PILOT
- Late relapses are possible with pegIFN treatments.

CO-PILOT and SOUND-C2
- PegIFN is able to achieve good SVR rates in difficult-to-treat patients, such as previous nonresponders (CO-PILOT) and patients who are cirrhotic (SOUND-C2).

AI444-040 trial
- Combination of an NS5B and an NS5A polymerase inhibitors lead to extermely high SVR rates in genotypes 1, 2, and 3.

at the end of treatment. Two genotype 1a patients relapsed: one at posttreatment week 8 and the other at posttreatment week 36. SVR12 and 24 rates were 91% and SVR36 rate was 82%. Resistance mutation analysis showed a D168V mutation for the first patient and a Y448H mutation for the second patient. Even if limited to 1 patient, this late relapse with a mutant clone is worrisome, especially considering that the Food and Drug Administration (FDA) now allows SVR12 as an end point for clinical trials.

The CO-PILOT study differed from PILOT, as it was for genotype 1 treatment-naïve and previous nonresponders to HCV treatment, without cirrhosis or bridging fibrosis.[17] It also used ABT-333, another non-nucleoside NS5B polymerase inhibitor, instead of ABT-072. There were 2 arms for naïve patients (ABT-450/r 250/100 mg every day (n = 19) versus 150/100 mg every day (n = 14) + ABT-333 and RBV) and 1 arm for nonresponders (ABT-450/r 150/100 mg every day + 333 400 + RBV; n = 17, including 11 partial responders and 6 null responders). All patients were treated for 12 weeks. SVR12 was achieved by 95% and 93% of the naïve patients and 47% of the nonresponders. Failure in the naive group was secondary to early discontinuation. For the nonresponders, there were 7 breakthroughs and 2 early relapses at week 2 posttreatment. Genotype 1a versus 1b and IL28B polymorphism did not affect the outcome in naïve patients. Interpretation is limited for the nonresponders, as there were no patients with a CC polymorphism and only 1 patient with genotype 1b.

The SOUND-C2 study from Boehringer Ingelheim had the peculiarity to have included patients with compensated cirrhosis.[18] The number of patients included is also impressive, with a total of 362. It is a phase IIb open-label trial for genotype 1 treatment-naïve patients. There were 5 arms using different combinations of BI201335, BI207127, and RBV. All patients received BI201335 120 mg every day and, except group 5, RBV. Group 1 was on BI201335, BI20127 600 mg 3 times a day, and RBV for 16 weeks, group 2 for 28 weeks, and group 3 for 40 weeks. Group 4 was on treatment for 28 weeks but with BI201227 600 mg twice a day and group 5 received only BI201335 and BI20127 600 mg 3 times a day without RBV for 28 weeks. The fifth group was stopped early by the FDA after the randomization of 46 patients. Overall, 59% of group 1, 61% of group 2, 68% of group 4, and 39% of group 5 achieved SVR12. As the treatment is longer for group 3, data are available only for post-treatment week 4 with 56% SVR4. SVR rates were higher for the patients with genotype 1b. IL28B affected the outcome of patients with genotype 1a (75% vs 32% for CC vs non-CC genotypes), but not genotype 1b (82% vs 84%). The subanalysis of patients with cirrhosis included 37 patients.[19] The combination of SVR12 for groups 1 and 2 and SVR4 for group 3 produced an SVR rate of 57% for the group on BI20127 3 times a day. The rates were 54% for group 4 and 33% for group 5. Again, genotype 1b was a good prognostic factor. Numbers were too small to analyze for IL28B polymorphism.

Bristol-Meyers Squibb and Gilead Sciences combined their drugs in the AI444-040 trial.[20] It was a study for genotype 1, 2, and 3 treatment-naïve patients. Currently, it is the only study to offer a pegIFN-free triple combination to genotype 2 and 3. Four of the 6 arms were dual therapy, combining daclatasvir and the nucleotide NS5B polymerase inhibitor GS-7977, but the last 2 arms also added RBV. Arms A, C, and E were for genotype 1 and arms B, D, and F for genotypes 2 and 3. Arms A and B used GS-7977 400 mg every day for 7 days, then added daclatasvir 60 mg up to week 24. Arms C, D, E, and F started both drugs on day 1 and arms E and F also started RBV. All patients had viral loads lower than the level of quantification at week 4. RBV did not affect the magnitude of viral decline. All the patients with genotype 1 achieved SVR4. Genotype 2 and 3 SVR4 rates were 88% for arm B, 100% for arm D, and 79% for arm F. One of the patients in arm B relapsed. Two patients were lost to follow-up in group F. All the other patients had viral loads lower than the level of quantification.

QUADRUPLE PEGIFN-FREE THERAPY

The only quadruple pegIFN-free study is the Gilead Sciences all-oral quad regimen (NCT01353248) (see **Fig. 1**A, **Table 1**).[21] It is a phase II study for genotype 1, treatment-naïve patients who are not cirrhotic. It combines GS-5885 (30 mg every day vs 90 mg every day), GS-9451, tegobuvir, and RBV for 24 weeks. For the GS-5885 90-mg every day arm, the patients who had a week 2 viral load less than 25 IU/mL from weeks 2 to 10 were re-randomized at week 12 to stop or continue until week 24. The results are still preliminary.

SUMMARY

At this point in HCV drug development, no drug is expected to be potent enough and to have a high enough barrier to resistance to be used in monotherapy. SVR results of pegIFN-containing quadruple therapy are very impressive and will probably be available sooner than pegIFN-free treatment. The AI447-011 trial has the potential to greatly modify the treatment outcomes in treatment-experienced patients. SVR rates in the quadruple treatment arm seem to be less influenced by factors such as IL28B polymorphisms or genotype 1a versus 1b. On the other hand, pegIFN-free treatments are clearly the goal that would allow treatment for more patients and with potentially fewer side effects. The results are promising even in patients with cirrhosis (SOUND-C2) or treatment-experienced patients (CO-PILOT). AI44-040, PILOT, and CO-PILOT studies had very high SVR rates in well-selected populations, but the overall SVR rates are still usually lower in these trials than those of the current standard of care for patients with HCV genotype 1 and trials with larger sample sizes, and multiple combinations are in process.

REFERENCES

1. Brok J, Gluud LL, Gluud C. Ribavirin monotherapy for chronic hepatitis C. Cochrane Database Syst Rev 2009;4:CD005527.
2. Forestier N, Reesink HW, Weegink CJ, et al. Antiviral activity of telaprevir (VX-950) and peginterferon alfa-2a in patients with hepatitis C. Hepatology 2007; 46:640–8.
3. Gane E, Stedman C, Anderson J, et al. PSI-7977 + Ribavirin in HCV genotype 1 null responders: results from the ELECTRON trial [54LB]. In: Program, Abstracts of the 19th Conference on Retroviruses and Opportunistic Infections. Seattle, March 5–8, 2012.
4. Rong L, Dahari H, Ribeiro RM, et al. Rapid emergence of protease inhibitor resistance in hepatitis C virus. Sci Transl Med 2010;2:30–2.
5. Zeuzem S, Asselah T, Angus P, et al. High sustained virologic response following interferon-free treatment of chronic HCV Gt1 infection for 4 weeks with HCV protease inhibitor BI201335, polymerase inhibitor BI207127 and ribavirin, followed by BI201335 and PegIFN/Ribavirin—the SOUND-C1 study. Hepatology 2011;54:486A–7A.
6. Gane E, Di Bisceglie A, Sulkowski M, et al. VX-222/Telaprevir in combination with peginterferon-alfa-2a and ribavirin in treatment-naïve genotype 1 HCV pateitns treated for 12 weeks: ZENITH Study, SVR12 Interim Analysis. In: 22nd Conference of the Asian Pacific Association for the Study of the Liver (APASL). Taipei, February 16–19, 2012.

7. Penney M, De Souza C, Seepersaud S, et al. All IL28B gentoypes have high SVR rates in patients treated with VX-222 in combination with telaprevir/perginterferon/ribavirin in the ZENITH study. J Hepatol 2012;56:S476–7.

8. Vertex announces 12-week on-treatment data and SVR4 from phase 2 study of interferon-free (All-Oral) treatment regimen of INCIVEK®, VX-222 and ribavirin in people with genotype 1 hepatitis C. Press release. Available at: http://investors.vrtx.com/releasedetail.cfm?ReleaseID=650944. Accessed July 28, 2012.

9. Zeuzem S, Buggisch P, Agarwal K, et al. The protease inhibitor, GS-9256, and non-nucleoside polymerase inhibitor tegobuvir alone, with ribavirin, or pegylated interferon plus ribavirin in hepatitis C. Hepatology 2012;55:749–58.

10. Lok AS, Gardiner DF, Lawitz E, et al. Preliminary study of two antiviral agents for hepatitis C genotype 1. N Engl J Med 2012;366:216–24.

11. Vierling J, Flamm S, Gordon S, et al. Efficacy of boceprevir in prior null responders to peginterferon/ribavirin: the PROVIDE study. Hepatology 2011;54:199A.

12. Berg T, McHutchison J, Adda N, et al. SVR with Telaprevir, Peginterferon Alfa-2A and Ribavirin in HCV patients with well-characterized prior null response, partial response, viral breakthrough or relapse after PR. J Hepatol 2010;52:S2.

13. Harrington PR, Zeng W, Naeger LK. Clinical relevance of detectable but not quantifiable hepatitis C virus RNA during boceprevir or telaprevir treatment. Hepatology 2012;55:1048–57.

14. Lok AS, Gardiner DF, Hezode C, et al. Confirmation that quadruple therapy with Daclatasvir (NS5A Inhibitor), Asunaprevir (NS3 Inhibitor) and Peginterferon/Ribavirin results in a high rate of SVR4 in HCV genotype 1 null responders. J Hepatol 2012;56:S557.

15. Gane E, Pockros S, Zeuzem S, et al. Interferon-free treatment with a combination of Mericitabine and Danoprevir/r with or without Ribavirin in treatment-naive HCV genotype 1-infected patients. J Hepatol 2012;56:S555–6.

16. Lawitz E, Poordad F, Kowdley K, et al. A 12-week interferon-free regimen of ABT-450/r, ABT-072, and Ribavirin was well tolerated and achieved sustained virologic response in 91% treatment-naive HCV IL28B-CC genotype-1-infected subjects. J Hepatol 2012;56:S7.

17. Poordad F, Lawitz E, Kowdley G, et al. 12-Week interferon-free regimen of ABT/r + ABT-333 + ribavirin achieved SVR12 in more than 90% of treatment-naive HCV genotype-1-infected subjects and 47% of previous non-responders. J Hepatol 2012;56:S549–50.

18. Zeuzem S, Soriano V, Asselah T, et al. SVR4 and SVR12 with an interferon-free regimen of BI201335 and BI207127, +/- Ribavirin, in treatment-naive patients with chronic genotype-1 HCV infection: interim results of SOUND-C2. J Hepatol 2012;56:S45.

19. Soriano V, Gane E, Angus P, et al. The efficacy and safety of the interferon-free combination of BI201335 and BI207127 in genotype 1 HCV patients with cirrhosis—interim analysis from SOUND-C2. J Hepatol 2012;56:S559.

20. Sulkowski M, Gardiner DF, Lawitz E, et al. Potent viral suppression with all-oral combination of daclatasvir (NS5A Inhibitor) and GS-7977 (NS5B Inhibitor), +/- ribavirin, in treatment-naive patients with chronic HCV GT 1, 2, or 3. J Hepatol 2012;56:S560.

21. Sulkowski M, Rodriguez-Torres M, Lawitz E, et al. High sustained virologic response rate in treatment-naive HCV genotype 1A and 1B patients treated for 12 weeks with an interferon-free all-oral quad regimen: interim results. J Hepatol 2012;56:S560.

Nucleoside/Nucleotide Analogue Polymerase Inhibitors in Development

Paul J. Pockros, MD

KEYWORDS

- Nucleoside/nucleotide analogue polymerase inhibitors • Hepatitis C • Mericitabine
- Sofosbuvir (GS-7977) • Interferon-free therapy

KEY POINTS

- Nucleoside/nucleotide analogue polymerase inhibitors (NPIs) are analogues of natural substrates that bind the active site of NS5B and terminate viral RNA chain generation.
- NPIs generally provide a high genetic barrier to resistance and are effective in all genotypes; however, they have been difficult to develop.
- Patients receiving triple therapy with mericitabine showed a 20% increase in virologic response over pegylated interferon α + ribavirin (RBV) alone; however, the overall sustained viral response (SVR) rate was suboptimal (56.8%), the regimen required 24 weeks rather than 12 weeks, and was sensitive to both IL28B polymorphisms and cirrhosis versus no cirrhosis.
- Sofosbuvir (GS-7977) is a potent, specific hepatitis C virus (HCV) nucleotide analogue that is safe and well tolerated in clinical studies, taken only once daily, with or without food, and has excellent antiviral activity with broad HCV genotype coverage.
- A promising small study performed with daclatasvir and GS-7977 suggested that this combination would be effective for 24 weeks without RBV, and would have equally high SVR rates in genotypes 1a and 1b, irrespective of IL28B alleles.
- INX-189 will join the league of several other compounds in this class that were halted in development because of unexpected toxicities that appeared in phase II trials.
- New nucleoside/nucleotide analogues such as sofosbuvir (GS-7977) show high antiviral activities that, together with their high genetic barrier to resistance, suggest that they are optimal backbone candidates for all-oral combination therapies.

BACKGROUND

Hepatitis C virus (HCV) replication is initiated by the formation of the replication complex, a highly structured association of HCV viral proteins and RNA, cellular proteins, and of rearranged intracellular lipid membranes derived from the endoplasmic

Division of Gastroenterology/Hepatology, Liver Disease Center, Scripps Clinic, 10666 North Torrey Pines Road, La Jolla, CA 92067, USA
E-mail address: pockros.paul@scrippshealth.org

Clin Liver Dis 17 (2013) 105–110
http://dx.doi.org/10.1016/j.cld.2012.09.007
1089-3261/13/$ – see front matter © 2013 Elsevier Inc. All rights reserved.

reticulum.[1] An important enzyme in HCV RNA replication is NS5B, an RNA-dependent RNA polymerase (**Fig. 1**) that catalyzes the synthesis of a complementary negative-strand RNA by using the positive-strand RNA genome as a template.[2] From this newly synthesized negative-strand RNA, numerous positive RNA strands are produced that serve as templates for further replication and polyprotein translation. There is poor fidelity of the NS5B enzyme, which often leads to errors in its RNA sequencing. This in turn, results in numerous different isolates that are generated during HCV replication in a given patient, termed HCV quasispecies.[3]

These compounds fall into 2 groups: nucleoside/nucleotide polymerase inhibitors (NPI) and nonnucleoside polymerase inhibitors (NNPI). The NPIs are analogues of natural substrates that bind the active site of NS5B and terminate viral RNA chain generation.[1] They generally provide a high genetic barrier to resistance and are effective in all genotypes; however, they have been difficult to develop and thus have had limited availability.[4] NNPIs bind to various allosteric sites, inducing conformational changes in the polymerase enzyme. They have been easier to develop because multiple target sites have been identified. However, they have only low-to-medium antiviral efficacy, have a low barrier to resistance, are HCV genotype-dependent and subset-dependent, and their efficacy is influenced by IL28B polymorphisms.[5] Examples of NPIs are valopicitabine (NM283), mericitabine (R7128), balapiravir (R1626), sofosbuvir (GS7977), GS-938, and IDX184 (**Table 1**). **Fig. 2** shows the structure of selected nucleoside and nonnucleoside inhibitors.

NUCLEOSIDE ANALOGUES

Mericitabine (RG7128) a diisobutyl ester prodrug of a cytosine nucleoside analogue that is a potent, selective and noncytotoxic HCV polymerase inhibitor. The drug is active against all HCV genotypes and has a high barrier to resistance. It has been shown to be safe and well tolerated. Interim results of phase II clinical trials in HCV genotype 1-infected, 2-infected, and 3-infected patients of R7128 in combination with pegylated interferon (PEF-IFN) and ribavirin (RBV) revealed sustained viral response (SVR) rates of

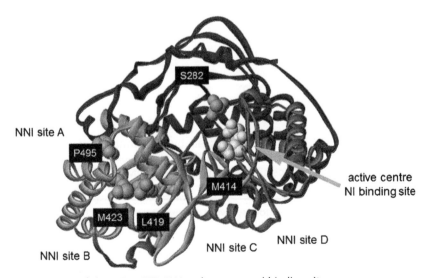

Fig. 1. Structure of the HCV NS5B RNA polymerase and binding sites.

Table 1
NS5B polymerase inhibitors

	Nucleoside/Nucleotide Analogue	Nonnucleoside/ Nonnucleotide Inhibitors
Approved	None	None
phase III	PSI-7977	ABT-333
		ABT-072
Phase II	M283 (Idenix; development halted because of toxicity)	
	R1626 (Roche; development halted because of toxicity)	
	Mericitabine (R7128; Genentech/Roche)	ANA-598
	PSI-938 (Pharmasett; development halted because	B120712
	of toxicity)	Filibur
	INX-189 (Inhibitex/BMS; development halted because	IDX-375
	of toxicity)	Tegobuvir
	ALS-2200/-2158 (Alios/Vertex)	VCH-916
		VX-222

mericitabine-based triple therapy compared with PegIFN-α alone.[6] The final results of patients in the triple therapy arm showed a 20% increase in virologic response over PegIFN + RBV alone, however the overall SVR rate was suboptimal (56.8%), the regimen required 24 weeks rather than 12 weeks, and was sensitive to both IL28B polymorphisms and cirrhosis versus no cirrhosis.[7]

In an all-oral regimen, with administration of mericitabine in combination with the protease inhibitor danoprevir (R7227/ITMN191) for 14 days, a synergistic antiviral activity of both drugs was observed.[8] However, in a longer study using this IFN-free combination for 12 or 24 weeks, viral breakthrough occurred in all patients unless they were treated for 24 weeks, and the regimen needed to include RBV.[9] The IFN-free combination was relatively effective in genotype 1b patients with an SVR of

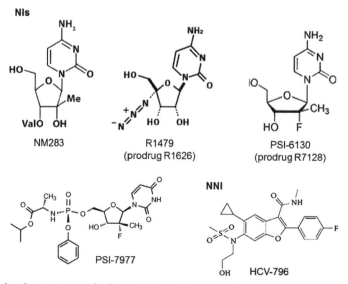

Fig. 2. Molecular structure of selected NS5B polymerase inhibitors.

71%; however, it was ineffective in genotype 1a (SVR 26%) and most of these treatment failures showed the most common resistant mutations to danoprevir (R155K, V36M/A, and D168T). One G1a patient had a virus with dual resistance to mericitabine and danoprevir, with mutations in NS5b (S282T) and NS3 (R155K). This combination regimen was deemed inadequate to move forward into development by itself, and is currently being studied in a quadruple combination with an NNPI (setrobuvir; ANA598-502).[10]

Promising clinical data have been published recently for sofosbuvir (GS-7977) a nucleoside analogue NS5B inhibitor effective against all HCV genotypes. Sofosbuvir (GS-7977) is a potent, specific HCV nucleotide analogue that is safe and well tolerated in clinical studies, taken only once daily, with or without food, and has excellent antiviral activity with broad HCV genotype coverage. Given as GS-7977 400 mg every day for 7 days in genotype 1, the monotherapy achieved a $4.7 \log_{10}$ reduction in viral load and showed a high barrier to resistance. No virologic breakthrough has been reported in any patient to date.

The PROTON study combined GS-7977 with PegIFN-α2a + RBV in arms with 200 mg or 400 mg of the drug + PegIFN-α2a + RBV for 12 weeks with an additional 12 weeks of PegIFN-α2a + RBV alone in patients with genotype 1, 2, and 3.[11] The interim analysis showed 100% SVR rates in the patients with genotype 2 and 3 with no viral breakthrough, relapse, or adverse events different from the PegIFN + RBV control arm.[12] The final results confirmed high SVR rates in genotype 1 with intention-to-treat SVR12 rates of 91% in the 400-mg arm and 88% in the 200-mg arm.[13] The combination regimen seemed to overcome IL28B genetic polymorphism predictors of poor response, with all 13/13 patients with TT allele achieving an SVR12. There were no viral breakthroughs observed on GS-7977 400 mg or during PEG/RBV. One relapse was observed 4 weeks after discontinuation and no late relapses (>+4 weeks to +24 weeks) were observed. There were no study drug discontinuations as a result of GS-7977-related adverse or serious adverse events, and no safety signal has been identified for GS-7977. S282T-resistant variants were not observed in any patient.[13]

In HCV genotype 2-infected and 3-infected patients, GS-7977 (400 mg once daily) in combination with RBV for 12 weeks + PegIFN-α for 4 to 12 weeks resulted in 100% rapid viral response and 100% week 12 SVR rates and GS-7977 + RBV alone achieved 100% SVR12 rates in 10 of 10 patients from New Zealand.[14] No GS-7977-associated side effects were reported, and no virologic breakthrough was observed. Further, the IFN-free arm showed the lessening impact on hemoglobin (Hgb) when just RBV+GS-7977 was given as the average Hgb reduction was 2 g or less. As well, there was no effect on absolute neutrophil count when PegIFN-α2a was not included in the regimen. This study changed the treatment paradigm for HCV in genotypes 2/3.

The ELECTRON study also evaluated this IFN-free regimen of GS-7977 400 mg once daily + RBV in 10 patients with genotype 1 who were previous null responders to PegIFN-α2a + RBV.[15] Most of the patients in this small trial were genotype 1a and had unfavorable IL28B allele types, and all of these patients relapsed when the 12-week oral regimen was completed. One patient with the IL28B CC allele had an SVR12. This study clearly showed that a more potent combination regimen is needed for genotype 1 null responders.

Results of the other 25 genotype 1 treatment-naive patients in the ELECTRON study treated with GS-7977 + RBV alone showed 88% SVR12 rates. However, a press release of the QUANTUM study genotype 1 treatment-naive data 24 weeks in a US population showed an SVR rate of only 53%.[16] At the time of this writing, we have no other information to explain the discrepancy between these 2 studies. However, it is likely that this regimen is not adequate for patients with genotype 1. A promising small study performed with daclatasvir and GS-7977 suggested that this combination would be effective for 24 weeks without RBV, and would have equally high SVR rates in genotypes 1a and 1b, irrespective of IL28B alleles.[17] Gilead Sciences has recently announced the initiation of a phase III study using their own NS5A inhibitor (GS-5885) + GS-7977 with or without RBV for 12 or 24 weeks.[18]

DRUG TOXICITIES

A striking example of this rapidly changing field was the announcement in August, 2012 that Bristol-Myers Squibb (BMS, New York, NY) voluntarily suspended an ongoing phase II study of BMS-986,094, which was formerly known as INX-189 (an NPI) after a patient who had received a 200-mg dose of the drug developed heart failure.[19] BMS had earlier purchased Inhibitex Pharmaceuticals (Alpharetta, GA) for $2.5 billion to combine the INX-189 with declatasvir, their NS5A inhibitor, as a regimen to compete with the GS-7977 + GS-5885 combination being studied by Gilead Sciences. INX-189 has now joined the league of other compounds in this class that were halted in development because of unexpected toxicities which appeared in phase II trials. These compounds include NM283 (Idenix, Cambridge, MA; development halted because of gastrointestinal toxicity), balapiravir [R1626] (Hoffmann-La Roche, Nutley, NJ; development halted because of lymphocytopenia), and PSI-938 (Pharmasett, Durham, NC; development halted because of hepatotoxicity). Thus, unexpected toxicities remain a risk for nucleoside analogues that have not yet been given to patients for at least 12 weeks, such as ALS-2200/-2158 (Alios, San Francisco, CA/Vertex, Cambridge, MA) and IDX-184 (Idenix, Cambridge, MA).

SUMMARY

New nucleoside/nucleotide analogues such as sofosbuvir (GS-7977) show high antiviral activities that, together with their high genetic barrier to resistance, suggest that they are optimal backbone candidates for all-oral combination therapies. Several trials are ongoing to further define the potential of all-oral regimens with sofosbuvir (GS-7977), including NS3 protease inhibitors, NS5A inhibitors, and RBV. Recent interim analyses indicate that many patients treated with only 2 direct-acting antiviral agents experience viral breakthrough, which can be significantly reduced by the addition of RBV without PegIFN-α.[20] It remains unclear if RBV will continue to be needed in a regimen combining 2 potent drugs, and early data suggest that it may not be.

REFERENCES

1. Moradpour D, Penin F, Rice CM. Replication of hepatitis C virus. Nat Rev Microbiol 2007;5:453–63.
2. Lesburg CA, Cable MB, Ferrari E, et al. Crystal structure of the RNA-dependent RNA polymerase from hepatitis C virus reveals a fully encircled active site. Nat Struct Biol 1999;6:937–43.
3. Mauss S, Berg T, Rockstroh J, et al. Short guide to hepatitis C. Germany: Flying Publisher & Kamps; 2012.
4. Koch U, Narjes F. Recent progress in the development of inhibitors of the hepatitis C virus RNA-dependent RNA polymerase. Curr Top Med Chem 2007;7:1302–29.
5. Sarrazin C, Zeuzem S. Resistance to direct antiviral agents in patients with hepatitis C virus infection. Gastroenterology 2010;138:447–62.
6. Pockros P, Jensen DM, Tsai N. First SVR data with the nucleoside analogue polymerase inhibitor mericitabine (RG7128) combined with peginterferon/ribavirin in

treatment-naive HCV G1/4 patients: interim analysis of the JUMP-C trial. J Hepatol 2011;54:538.

7. Pockros P, Jensen D, Tsai N, et al. SVR-12 among G1/4 treatment-naïve patients receiving mericitabine in combination with PEG-IFNα-2A/RBV: interim analysis from the Jump-C study. J Hepatol 2012;56(Suppl 2):S477.

8. Gane EJ, Roberts SK, Stedman CA, et al. Oral combination therapy with a nucleoside polymerase inhibitor (RG7128) and danoprevir for chronic hepatitis C genotype 1 infection (INFORM-1): a randomised, double-blind, placebo-controlled, dose-escalation trial. Lancet 2010;376:1467–75.

9. Gane EJ, Pockros P, Zeuzem S, et al. Interferon-free treatment with a combination of mericitabine and danoprevir/R with or without ribavirin in treatment-naïve HCV genotype 1-infected patients. J Hepatol 2012;56(Suppl 2):S555.

10. Hoffmann-La Roche. ANNAPURNA: A study of the combination of RO5466731, RO5190591, ritonavir and Copegus (ribavirin) with or without RO5024048 in patients with chronic hepatitis C who are either treatment-naive or have previously experienced a null response to interferon-based treatment [ClinicalTrials.gov identifier NCT01628094]. US National Institutes of Health, ClinicalTrials.gov [online]. Available at: http://www.clinicaltrials.gov. Accessed August 26, 2012.

11. Nelson DR, Lalezari J, Lawitz E, et al. Once daily PSI-7977 plus PEG-IFN/RBV in HCV GT1: 98% rapid virologic response, complete early virologic response: the PROTON study [abstract 1372]. J Hepatol 2011;54(Suppl 1):S544.

12. Lalezari J, Lawitz E, Rodriguez-Torres M, et al. Once daily PSI-7977 plus PEGIFN/RBV in a phase 2B trial: rapid virologic suppression in treatment-naïve patients with HCV GT2/GT3 [abstract 61]. J Hepatol 2011;54(Suppl 1):S28.

13. Lawitz E, Lalezari JP, Hassanein T, et al. Once-daily PSI-7977 plus peg/RBV in treatment-naive patients with HCV GT1: robust end of treatment response rates are sustained post-treatment. Hepatology 2011;54:113.

14. Gane EJ, Stedman CA, Hyland RH, et al. PSI-7977: ELECTRON interferon is not required for sustained virologic response in treatment-naïve patients with HCV GT2 or GT3. 62nd Annual Meeting of the American Association for the Study of Liver Diseases. San Francisco, November 4–8, 2011.

15. Gane EJ, Stedman C, Anderson J, et al. 100% rapid virologic response for PSI-7977 + ribavirin in genotype 1 null responders (ELECTRON): early viral decline similar to that observed in genotype 1 and genotype 2/3 treatment-naïve patients [abstract 54LB]. 19th Conference on Retroviruses and Opportunistic Infections. March 5–8, 2012.

16. Gilead announces early sustained virologic response rates for GS-7977 plus ribavirin in genotype 1 treatment-naïve hepatitis C patients–interim results reported from ELECTRON and QUANTUM studies. Barcelona (Spain): Gilead Sciences; 2012.

17. Sulkowski M, Gardiner D, Lawitz E, et al. Potent viral suppression with all-oral combination of daclatasvir (NS5A inhibitor) and GS-7977 (NS5B inhibitor), +/- ribavirin, in treatment-naïve patients with chronic HCV GT1, 2, or 3 [LB abstract 1422]. 47th Annual Meeting of the European Association for the Study of the Liver. Barcelona, April 18–22, 2012.

18. Available at: http://www.clinicaltrials.gov: Hepatitis C and Gilead Sciences. 2012. Accessed 12 October, 2012.

19. Pollack A. Bristol-Myers to suspend a drug study. New York, NY: The New York Times; 2012.

20. Zeuzem S, Buggisch P, Agarwal K, et al. The protease inhibitor GS-9256 and non-nucleoside polymerase inhibitor tegobuvir alone, with RBV or peginterferon plus RBV in hepatitis C. Hepatology 2012;55(3):749–58.

HCV NS5A Inhibitors in Development

Anna Suk-Fong Lok, MD

KEYWORDS

- Hepatitis C • Direct-acting antiviral agents • Daclatasvir • Asunaprevir • GS-7977
- Pegylated interferon • Ribavirin

KEY POINTS

- NS5A protein plays a key role in hepatitis C virus (HCV) replication.
- Daclatasvir is a first-in-class inhibitor of HCV NS5A replication complex with potent antiviral activity but low barrier to resistance.
- Daclatasvir as triple therapy in combination with pegylated interferon and ribavirin results in a high rate of early virologic response in treatment-naïve patients with genotype 1 infection, and preliminary data suggest a high rate of sustained virologic response.
- Daclatasvir as quadruple therapy in combination with asunaprevir, pegylated interferon, and ribavirin results in a high rate of sustained virologic response in genotype 1 prior null responders.
- Daclatasvir as dual therapy with GS-7977 results in a high rate of sustained virologic response in treatment-naïve patients with genotype 1, 2, or 3 infections.
- Daclatasvir as dual therapy with asunaprevir results in a high rate of sustained virologic response in genotype 1b prior null responders.

INTRODUCTION

Improvement in the understanding of hepatitis C virus (HCV) biology and the availability of in vitro models to study HCV replication in the past decade have facilitated the development of direct-acting antiviral agents (DAAs) that target specific steps in the HCV

The author is advisor to Achillon, Astex, Bristol-Myers Squibb, GlaxoSmithKline, Janssen, and Roche.

Financial disclosures: The author has received research grants from Abbott, Bristol-Myers Squibb, Gilead, GlaxoSmithKline, Merck, and Roche.

Daclatasvir and other NS5A inhibitors mentioned in this article as well as asunaprevir and GS-7977 are investigational drugs and have not been approved by the FDA for treatment of hepatitis C.

Division of Gastroenterology and Hepatology, University of Michigan Health System, University of Michigan, 1500 East Medical Center Drive, 3912 Taubman Center, SPC 5362, Ann Arbor, MI 48109, USA

E-mail address: aslok@umich.edu

http://dx.doi.org/10.1016/j.cld.2012.09.006
1089-3261/13/$ – see front matter © 2013 Elsevier Inc. All rights reserved.

liver.theclinics.com

replication cycle. DAAs have potent antiviral activity but they select for antiviral drug resistance variants. Virologic breakthrough and the emergence of resistance-associated variants (RAVs) can occur within 3 days of DAA monotherapy. Virologic response can be improved and drug resistance minimized when DAAs are used in combination with pegylated interferon alfa (PEG-IFNα) and ribavirin (RBV) or when DAAs with different viral targets are used in combination. Currently, there are 3 classes of DAAs in clinical trials: NS3/4A protease inhibitors, NS5A replication complex inhibitors, and NS5B polymerase inhibitors. NS5B polymerase inhibitors can be further divided into nucleos/tide inhibitors and non-nucleoside/nucleotide inhibitors.

In 2011, 2 protease inhibitors, telaprevir and boceprevir, were approved for the treatment of genotype (GT) 1 HCV infection. These drugs used as triple therapy in combination with PEG-IFNα and RBV resulted in significant improvement in the rate of sustained virologic response (SVR), with SVR rates of 67% to 75% in treatment-naïve patients[1,2] but only 29% to 40% in patients who had a null response to prior treatment with PEG-IFNα and RBV.[3,4] Although the addition of telaprevir and boceprevir to PEG-IFNα and RBV therapy improved the virologic response, these drugs also increased the complexity of the treatment regimen and the occurrence of adverse events. Furthermore, RAVs were detected in approximately 50% of patients who failed to achieve SVR. Therefore, there is a need to develop other DAAs, particular DAAs with other viral targets.

NS5A AS A TARGET FOR DAA

HCV NS5A is a 447 amino acid (aa) phosphoprotein. It does not possess any enzymatic activity, but it has a crucial role in HCV replication. NS5A is comprised of 3 distinct structural domains as well as an amphipathic α–helix at its N terminus that functions in membrane localization.[5] Domain I (aa 37–213) is essential for viral RNA replication and has been crystallized as a homodimer. Domains II (aa 250–342) and III (aa 356–447) are less well characterized. Domain II is involved with binding to cyclophilin A and has been postulated to play a role in antagonizing the innate immune response to HCV. Domain III seems to be important for the assembly of infectious viral particles. Because NS5A is involved in multiple steps in HCV replication, inhibitors of NS5A may have potent antiviral activity.

DACLATASVIR
Overview

Daclatasvir (BMS-790052, DCV) is the first-in-class HCV NS5A inhibitor. In vitro studies showed that it is highly potent with picomolar half-maximum effective concentrations in replicons expressing a broad range of HCV GTs with higher activity against GT1b compared with GT1a and lower activity against GT2 and GT3.[6] DCV displays a high therapeutic index and is specific for HCV; however, it has a low barrier to resistance. In vitro and clinical studies showed that RAVs can be readily selected, more so for GT1a isolates than GT1b isolates. The most common substitutions are located at residues 28, 30, 31, and 93 for GT1a and residues 31 and 93 for GT1b.[7] Single substitutions in GT1a isolates can confer more than 1000-fold resistance, whereas single substitutions in GT1b isolates generally confer less than 50-fold resistance. A combination of substitutions (eg, at residues 30 and 93 or 31 and 93) increases resistance markedly. The location of the resistance substitutions suggests that DCV targets domain I of NS5A.

Multiple ascending dose studies in humans showed that the mean terminal half-life of DCV was 12 to 15 hours supporting once-daily dosing.[8] Dosages of 1 to 100 mg daily administered for 14 days were well tolerated. Dosages of 10, 20, and 60 mg daily were tested in phase II trials, with better responses at 60-mg dosages. DCV is a substrate of cytochrome P450 3A4 and of P-glycoprotein and has the potential for drug-drug interactions similar to telaprevir and boceprevir. Studies have shown that there is no drug interaction between DCV and asunaprevir (ASV, BMS-650032, NS3/4A protease inhibitor) and GS-7977 (NS5B nucleotide polymerase inhibitor with pan-genotypic activity). DCV has also been shown to have no interaction with combined oral contraceptives.[9] Pharmacokinetic studies in patients with severe hepatic impairment suggest that dose adjustment is not required in patients with cirrhosis, including those with Child C cirrhosis.[10]

DCV has been studied in IFN-containing regimens and in IFN-free regimens and in treatment-naïve as well as in treatment-experienced patients.

IFN-Containing Regimens

DCV has been studied as a triple therapy in combination with PEG-IFNα and RBV in treatment-naïve and in treatment-experienced patients and as a quadruple therapy in combination with ASV, PEG-IFNα, and RBV in patients who were null responders (<2 log decrease in HCV RNA after ≥12 weeks of treatment) to prior PEG-IFNα and RBV therapy.

Triple therapy of DCV, PEG-IFNα, and RBV

GT1b treatment-naïve Japanese patients In a study by Suzuki and colleagues,[11] 27 treatment-naïve GT1b Japanese patients were randomized to receive DCV 10 mg (n = 9), 60 mg (n = 10), or placebo (n = 8) and PEG-IFNα-2b + RBV. Patients in the 2 DCV groups who had a protocol-defined response (PDR) based on HCV RNA less than limit of quantification (LOQ) at week 4 and HCV RNA less than limit of detection (LOD) at week 12 continued triple therapy until week 24, whereas those who failed to achieve PDR continued triple therapy until week 48. All patients in the placebo group continued PEG-IFNα and RBV until week 48. The rates of rapid virologic response (RVR, HCV RNA less than LOD at week 4) were 78%, 80%, and 0%; extended RVR (eRVR, HCV RNA less than LOD at week 4 and week 12) rates were 67%, 80%, and 0%; and PDR rates were 78%, 100%, and 0% for the groups that received DCV 10 mg, DCV 60 mg, or placebo, respectively. Among the 17 DCV recipients who achieved PDR, 16 had an end of treatment response (EOTR) at week 24 and 15 had SVR$_{24}$. A similar study by Izumi and colleagues[12] used PEG-IFNα-2a with 9, 8, and 8 patients in the groups that received DCV 10 mg, DCV 60 mg, and placebo. Rates of RVR were 78%, 63%, and 13% and eRVR rates were 67%, 63%, and 13%, respectively, in the 3 treatment groups. Fifteen out of 17 DCV recipients achieved PDR and all 15 had EOTR and SVR$_{24}$.

When the results of these 2 studies were combined, PDR was achieved in 78% and 100% of patients who received DCV 10 mg and DCV 60 mg, respectively; among those who achieved PDR, 93% and 94% patients, respectively, achieved SVR$_{24}$ after 24 weeks of triple therapy. In both studies, adverse events in the triple-therapy groups were similar to those who received dual therapy with PEG-IFNα and RBV. These data support the development of DCV as triple therapy with PEG-IFNα and RBV in treatment-naïve GT1b patients and the use of 60-mg doses of DCV going forward.

GT1b nonresponder Japanese patients In Suzuki and colleagues'[11] study mentioned earlier, 18 patients (9 null responders and 9 partial responders), with only 1 having the IL28B rs12979860 CC, were randomized to receive DCV 10 mg or 60 mg (n = 9 in each group) in combination with PEG-IFNα-2b and RBV. Rates of RVR were 56%

and 33%; eRVR 56% and 22%; and PDR 56% and 33% for the groups that received DCV 10 mg and 60 mg, respectively. All 8 patients who achieved PDR had EOTR but only 4 achieved SVR_{24}. In Izumi and colleagues'[12] study, 17 patients (12 null responders and 5 partial responders) with none having IL28B rs12979860 CC were randomized to receive DCV 10 mg (n = 8) or 60 mg (n = 9) in combination with PEG-IFNα-2a and RBV. Rates of RVR were 63% and 89%; eRVR 63% and 78%; and PDR 88% and 78%. All 14 patients who achieved PDR had an EOTR response but only 10 achieved SVR_{24}.

When the results of these two studies were combined, PDR was achieved in 71% and 56% of patients who received DCV 10 mg and DCV 60 mg, respectively; among those who achieved PDR, 50% and 80% patients, respectively, achieved SVR_{24} after 24 weeks of triple therapy. In both studies, NS5A RAVs were detected in all patients with treatment failure (10 virologic breakthrough and 8 relapse). These data indicate that DCV as triple therapy is inadequate in patients with a prior partial or null response to PEG-IFNα and RBV.

GT1 and GT4 treatment-naïve US and European patients (COMMAND-1 study) In a study by Hezode and colleagues,[13] 365 patients with GT1 (72%–78% GT1a) and 30 with GT4 infection in the United States and Europe were randomized to receive DCV 20 mg, 60 mg, or placebo (2:2:1) in combination with PEG-IFNα and RBV. Cirrhosis was present in 5% to 10% of patients and 28% to 33% had IL28B rs12979860 CC. Patients in the DCV groups who had PDR based on HCV RNA less than LOQ at week 4 and less than LOD at week 10 were randomized at the end of week 12 to continue triple therapy until week 24 or to stop DCV and continue PEG-IFNα + RBV to week 24. Patients in the DCV groups who failed to achieve PDR and all patients in the placebo group continued treatment with PEG-IFNα + RBV from week 13 to week 48. Among the patients with GT1, rates of RVR were 60%, 57%, and 15%; and eRVR rates were 54%, 54%, and 14% in the groups that received DCV 20 mg, DCV 60 mg, and placebo, respectively. PDR was achieved in 71% and 72% of patients in the DCV 20-mg and DCV 60-mg groups, respectively. Among the patients who achieved PDR, the EOTR at week 24 was observed in 96% and 94% of patients in the DCV 20-mg and DCV 60-mg groups who stopped DCV at week 12 and in 88% and 100% of those who continued DCV until week 24.

Of the 30 patients with GT4 infection, undetectable HCV RNA at week 4 was achieved in 3 out of 12, 4 out of 12, and 0 out of 6 and at week 12 in 7 out of 12, 12 out of 12, and 3 out of 6 patients in the groups that received DCV 20 mg, DCV 60 mg, and placebo, respectively.

Adverse events were similar across the 3 groups, except for nausea and dry skin, which were reported by a higher percent of patients in the DCV groups. The frequency of grade 3 or 4 changes in blood counts, alanine aminotransferase (ALT), and total bilirubin were similar in the 3 groups.

These data showed that DCV as triple therapy with PEG-IFNα and RBV in treatment-naïve GT1 (predominantly GT1a) US and European patients resulted in high rates of early virologic responses. Treatment was well tolerated, but further follow-up is necessary to determine the rate of SVR in these patients, particularly those with GT1a infection or unfavorable IL28B genotype.

GT1 null and partial responder US and European patients (COMMAND-2 trial) In a study by Ratziu and colleagues,[14] US and European patients with GT1 (41%–71% GT1a) infection and a null or partial response to prior PEG-IFNα + RBV therapy were randomized to DCV 20 mg (n = 203), DCV 60 mg (n = 199), or placebo (n = 17) in combination with PEG-IFNα and RBV. Cirrhosis was present in 13% to 21%

of patients and 88% to 94% had IL28B rs12979860 CT/TT. Patients in the DCV groups who achieved PDR (HCV RNA less than LOQ at week 4 and less than LOD at week 12) were randomized to stop all drugs at week 24 or to stop DCV and continue PEG-IFNα and RBV until week 48. Patients in the DCV groups who did not achieve PDR stopped DCV at week 24; these patients and all those in the placebo group continued PEG-IFNα and RBV until week 48. On-treatment responses up to week 12 were presented. Rates of RVR were 21%, 21%, and 0%; eRVR rates were 18%, 20%, and 0%; and PDR rates were 25%, 30%, 0% for null responders who received DCV 20 mg, DCV 60 mg, and placebo, respectively. For partial responders, rates of RVR were 26%, 39%, and 0%; eRVR rates were 26%, 36%, and 0%; and PDR rates were 37%, 52%, and 0%, respectively. Although the final results are not yet available, data to date indicate that triple therapy with DCV, PEG-IFNα, and RBV are inadequate for most patients with GT1 and a null or a partial response to PEG-IFNα and RBV.

Quadruple therapy with DCV, ASV, PEG-IFNα, and RBV

GT1 null responder US and European patients In a study by Lok and colleagues,[15] 21 US patients without cirrhosis with GT1 infection with a null response to prior PEG-IFNα and RBV therapy were enrolled in the sentinel cohort and randomized to receive quadruple therapy with DCV 60 mg daily, ASV 600 mg twice daily, PEG-IFNα and RBV or dual therapy with DCV and ASV for 24 weeks. Among the 10 patients in the quadruple therapy group, 9 had GT1a infection and 9 had IL28B rs12979860 CT/TT. All 10 patients achieved EOTR as well as SVR_{12} (**Fig. 1**). Nine patients had SVR_{24} and 9 had SVR_{48}. HCV RNA was detectable but less than LOQ in 1 patient at posttreatment week 24 and in another patient at posttreatment week 48, both patients had undetectable HCV RNA on retesting. Quadruple therapy was well tolerated; the most common adverse events were diarrhea and transient elevation in ALT, both of which were attributed to ASV.

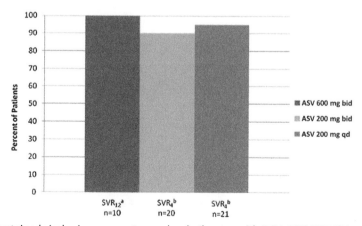

Fig. 1. Sustained virologic response to quadruple therapy with DCV, ASV, PEG-IFNα, and RBV in GT1 null responder US and European patients. All patients received DCV 60 mg daily and standard dosages of PEG-IFNα and RBV. Dosages of ASV varied from 600 mg twice daily to 200 mg every day. (*Data from* [a] Lok AS, Gardiner DF, Lawitz E, et al. Preliminary study of two antiviral agents for hepatitis C genotype 1. N Engl J Med 2012;366:216–24; and [b] Lok AS, Gardiner DF, Hezode C, et al. Confirmation that quadruple therapy with daclatasvir (NS5A Inhibitor), asunaprevir (NS3 Inhibitor) and peginterferon/ribavirin results in high rate of SVR4 in HCV genotype 1 null responders. J Hepatol 2012;56(Suppl 2):S557.)

Preliminary data from 41 (88% GT1a, 100% IL28B rs12979860 CT/TT) US and European patients in the expanded cohort who received quadruple therapy at a lower dose of ASV, 200 mg daily (n = 21) or ASV 200 mg twice daily (n = 20) showed that EOTR was achieved in 100% and 90% patients and SVR$_4$ in 95% and 90%, respectively, in the two groups (see **Fig. 1**).[16] These data confirmed that 24 weeks of quadruple therapy with DCV, ASV, PEG-IFNα, and RBV achieves a very high rate of SVR (>90%), even in the most difficult to treat patients, predominantly GT1a, unfavorable IL28B prior null responders. However, this approach is feasible only for patients who can tolerate PEG-IFNα and RBV, and response rates are likely lower and adverse event rates higher for patients with cirrhosis.

IFN-FREE REGIMENS
Dual or Triple Therapy with DCV + GS-7977 ± RBV

GT1/2/3 treatment-naïve US and European patients
In a study by Sulkowski and colleagues,[17] treatment-naïve US and European patients without cirrhosis with GT1, 2, or 3 infection were randomized to receive a combination of DCV 60 mg daily and GS-7977 400 mg daily, with or without RBV for 24 weeks. Half of the patients who received dual therapy received lead-in GS-7977 monotherapy for 7 days. Randomization was stratified for HCV genotype: 1 versus 2/3. Among the patients with GT1 infection, 71% to 73% had GT1a. Across all groups, IL28B rs12979860 CC was present in 27% to 57% of patients. Virologic response was similar across all 3 treatment groups regardless of HCV or IL28B genotype. For the 44 patients with GT1 infection, the rates of EOTR were 87%, 86%, and 93% (lower rate of EOTR compared with SVR$_4$ because missing values were considered as treatment failure), and the SVR$_4$ rates were 100%, 100%, and 100% for the groups that received dual therapy with or without GS-7977 lead-in and triple therapy with RBV, respectively (**Fig. 2**). EOTR rates for the 3 treatment groups among patients with GT2/3 infection

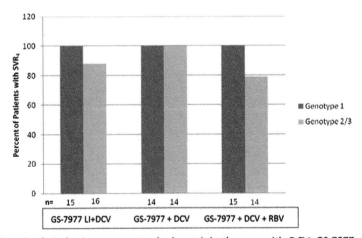

Fig. 2. Sustained virologic response to dual or triple therapy with DCV, GS-7977 ± RBV in GT1/2/3 treatment-naïve US or European patients. Treatment was administered for 24 weeks. LI, 7-day lead-in therapy with GS-7977. (*Data from* Sulkowski MS, Gardiner DF, Lawitz F, et al. Potent viral suppression with all-oral combination of Daclatasvir (NS5A Inhibitor) and GS-7977 (NS5B Inhibitor) +/- ribavirin, in treatment-naive patients with chronic HCV GT1, 2, or 3. J Hepatol 2012;56(Suppl 2):S560.)

were 93%, 93%, and 86%, and SVR_4 rates 88%, 100%, and 79%, respectively. Treatment was well tolerated; the most common adverse events were fatigue, headache, and nausea. Grade 3/4 elevations of ALT and bilirubin were not observed, and the only major change in blood counts was anemia, which occurred only in patients who received ribavirin. These data suggest that 24 weeks of dual therapy with DCV and GS-7977 can result in very high rates of SVR in treatment-naïve patients without cirrhosis with GT1, 2, or 3 infections and the addition of RBV did not confer any benefit.

Dual Therapy with DCV and ASV

GT1 null responder US and European patients

In the study by Lok and colleagues[15] mentioned earlier, 11 US patients without cirrhosis with GT1 infection (9 GT1a, 10 IL28B rs12979860 CT/TT) and a null response to prior therapy with PEG-IFNα and RBV were randomized to receive dual therapy with DCV and ASV for 24 weeks. HCV RNA levels declined rapidly in all patients during the first week and 7 (64%) patients achieved RVR; however, 6 patients experienced virologic breakthrough. The remaining 5 patients achieved EOTR, but one relapsed and only 4 (2/2 GT1b and 2/9 GT1a) patients achieved SVR_4 **(Fig. 3)**. These 4 patients maintained SVR up to the last visit, 48 weeks after the completion of treatment.

PEG-IFNα and RBV was added as rescue therapy in the 6 patients with virologic breakthrough. Two patients had a decline in HCV RNA levels but remained viremic. The remaining 4 patients achieved EOTR but only 2 achieved SVR.

All 6 patients with virologic breakthrough had RAVs in both the NS5A domain (Q30R, L31M/V, and Y93C/N) and the NS3 protease domain (R155K and D168A/E/T/V/Y). The patient with viral relapse had preexistence of the NS3 protease resistance variant

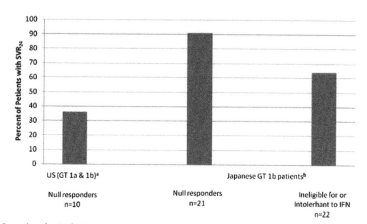

Fig. 3. Sustained virologic response to dual therapy with DCV and ASV in GT1 US and Japanese patients. All patients received DCV 60 mg daily. The 10 US patients and the first 10 Japanese null responders received ASV 600 mg twice daily, whereas the remaining Japanese patients received ASV 200 mg twice daily. (*Data from* [a] Lok AS, Gardiner DF, Lawitz E, et al. Preliminary study of two antiviral agents for hepatitis C genotype 1. N Engl J Med 2012;366:216–24; and [b] Suzuki F, Ikeda K, Toyota J, et al. Dual oral therapy with the NS5A inhibitor daclatasvir (BMS-790052) and NS3 protease inhibitor asunaprevir (BMS-650032) in HCV genotype 1B-infected null responders or ineligible/intolerant to peginterferon/ribavirin. J Hepatol 2012;56(Suppl 2):S7–8.)

R155K at baseline that was also present at the time of viral relapse, whereas the NS5A resistance variant Q30E was detected only at relapse.

These data provided the proof of concept that SVR can be achieved with combination DAAs in the absence of PEG-IFNα and RBV. Response in patients without cirrhosis with GT1b infection was encouraging, but dual therapy with DCV and ASV is inadequate for most patients with GT1a infection, which is likely related to the lower barrier to resistance to both drugs. These results highlight the importance of selecting appropriate DAAs in IFN-free combination DAA regimens to prevent multidrug resistance. Further study is ongoing to confirm the role of dual therapy with DCV and ASV in US and European patients with GT1b infection and a null response to prior PEG-IFNα and RBV therapy.

GT1b Japanese patients with prior null response or who are ineligible for or intolerant to PEG-IFNα/RBV

In a pilot study by Chayama and colleagues,[18] 10 Japanese patients with GT1b infection and a null response to prior PEG-IFNα and RBV received 24 weeks of dual therapy with DCV and ASV (600 mg twice daily). Nine patients achieved EOTR as well as SVR_{24}. The remaining patient discontinued treatment at week 2 because of adverse events and had undetectable HCV RNA at the end of treatment and 24 weeks after stopping treatment. This study had been expanded to include 11 additional null responders and 22 patients who were ineligible for IFN-based regimens because of medical reasons (n = 18) or who discontinued PEG-IFNα and RBV therapy after less than 12 weeks of treatment because of intolerance (n = 4).[19] A lower dosage of ASV, 200 mg twice daily, was used. The rates of EOTR were 91% and 86%, and the rates for SVR_{24} were 91% and 64% in patients with a prior null response (including the 10 patients previously reported) and those who were ineligible for or intolerant to PEG-IFNα and RBV, respectively (see **Fig. 3**). Factors associated with treatment failure included preexisting NS5A RAV and inadequate drug exposure. Ten (23%) patients had baseline NS5A RAV Y93H; of these, only 5 achieved SVR. Most patients with virologic breakthrough or relapse had trough DCV and ASV plasma concentrations lower than the median for all patients. Data from this study showed that dual therapy with DCV and ASV can achieve a very high rate of SVR in Japanese patients with GT1b infection and a null response to prior therapy. The lower rate of SVR among patients ineligible for or intolerant to PEG-IFNα and RBV was surprising and may be related to poor adherence to medications as reflected by lower drug concentrations.

OTHER NS5A INHIBITORS
Other NS5A Inhibitors in Clinical Trials

Table 1 lists other NS5A inhibitors in clinical trials. Some of these new drugs are being tested as monotherapy in phase I dose-finding studies. ABT-267, GS-5885, and GSK-2336805 are also being tested as triple therapy in combination with PEG-IFNα and RBV or as quadruple therapy in combination with other DAAs and RBV. Very few patients have been enrolled into these studies, and only SVR data on subsets of patients have been presented. These drugs have the same resistance profile as DCV.

Second-Generation NS5A Inhibitors

Second-generation NS5A inhibitors have been developed, including MK-8742 and ACH-3102.[20,21] In vitro studies showed that RAVs to DCV confer lower resistance to these new compounds, whether this will translate into a higher barrier to resistance in vivo remains to be determined.

Table 1
Clinical trials of HCV NS5A inhibitors

Company	Drug	Trial Phase	HCV Genotype	Patient Population	Trial Design
Bristol-Myers Squibb	DCV (BMS-790052)	II/III	1, 2, 3, 4	Treatment naïve, nonresponder to PEG-IFN/RBV with or without protease inhibitor	Dual therapy with ASV (NS3) or GS-7977 (NS5B) Triple therapy with ASV (NS3) or GS-7977 (NS5B) and RBV Triple therapy with PEG-IFN or PEG-IFN and RBV Quadruple therapy with PEG-IFN or PEG-IFN and RBV
Abbott	ABT-267	I/II	1	Treatment naïve	Triple therapy with PEG-IFN/RBV Quadruple therapy with ABT-450r (NS3 with ritonavir boost) + ABT-333 (NS5B NNI) + RBV
Gilead	GS-5885	I/II	1	Treatment naïve	Triple or quadruple therapy with PEG-IFN/RBV + GS-9451 (NS3) Quadruple therapy with GS-9451 (NS3) + GS-9190 (NS5B NNI) + RBV
GlaxoSmithKline	GSK-2336805	I/II	1, 4	Treatment naïve	Monotherapy Triple therapy with PEG-IFN/RBV
Presidio	PPI-668	I	1	Treatment naïve	Monotherapy
Idenix	IDX-719	I/II	1	Treatment naïve	Monotherapy
Janssen	JNJ-47910382	I	1	Asian, treatment naïve	Monotherapy

Data from Available at: www.clinicaltrials.gov. Accessed July 1, 2012.

REFERENCES

1. Jacobson IM, McHutchison JG, Dusheiko G, et al. Telaprevir for previously untreated chronic hepatitis C virus infection. N Engl J Med 2011;364:2405–16.
2. Poordad F, McCone J Jr, Bacon BR, et al. Boceprevir for untreated chronic HCV genotype 1 infection. N Engl J Med 2011;364:1195–206.
3. Zeuzem S, Andreone P, Pol S, et al. Telaprevir for retreatment of HCV infection. N Engl J Med 2011;364:2417–28.
4. Bronowicki JP, Lencioni R, Marrero J, et al. Sustained virologic response (SVR) in prior peginterferon/ribavirin (PR) treatment failures after retreatment with boceprevir (BOC)-+-PR: the PROVIDE study interim results. J Hepatol 2012;54:S6.

5. Fridell RA, Qiu D, Wang C, et al. Resistance analysis of the hepatitis C virus NS5A inhibitor BMS-790052 in an in vitro replicon system. Antimicrob Agents Chemother 2010;54:3641–50.

6. Gao M, Nettles RE, Belema M, et al. Chemical genetics strategy identifies an HCV NS5A inhibitor with a potent clinical effect. Nature 2010;465:96–100.

7. Fridell RA, Wang C, Sun JH, et al. Genotypic and phenotypic analysis of variants resistant to hepatitis C virus nonstructural protein 5A replication complex inhibitor BMS-790052 in humans: in vitro and in vivo correlations. Hepatology 2011;54:1924–35.

8. Nettles RE, Gao M, Bifano M, et al. Multiple ascending dose study of BMS-790052, a nonstructural protein 5A replication complex inhibitor, in patients infected with hepatitis C virus genotype 1. Hepatology 2011;54:1956–65.

9. Bifano M, Sevinsky H, Persson A, et al. BMS-790052 has no effect on the pharmacokinetics of a combined oral contraceptive containing ethinyl estradiol and norgestimate in healthy female subjects. Hepatology 2011;54:991A–2A.

10. Bifano M, Sevinsky H, Persson A, et al. Single-dose pharmacokinetics of BMS-790052 in subjects with hepatic impairment compared with healthy subjects. Hepatology 2011;54:1004A.

11. Suzuki F, Chayama K, Kawakami Y, et al. BMS-790052, an NS5A replication complex inhibitor, in combination with peginterferon alpha-2b and ribavirin in Japanese treatment-naive and nonresponder patients with chronic HCV genotype 1 infection. Hepatology 2011;54:1441A.

12. Izumi N, Asahina Y, Yokosuka O, et al. Combination therapy of treatment-naive and nonresponder patients with HCV genotypoe1 infection with BMS-790052, an NS5A replication complex inhibitor, in combination with peginterferon alfa-2a and ribavirin. Hepatology 2011;54:1439A–40A.

13. Hezode C, Hirschfield G, Ghesquiere W, et al. BMS-790052, A NS5A replication complex inhibitor, combined with peginterferon alfa-2a and ribavirin in treatment-naive HCV-genotype 1 or 4 patients: phase 2B AI444010 study interim week 12 results. Hepatology 2011;54:474A–5A.

14. Ratziu V, Gadano S, Pol C, et al. Triple therapy with daclatasvir (DCV; BMS-790052), peginterferon alfa-2a and ribavirin in HCV-infected prior null and partial responders: 12-week results of phase 2B COMMAND-2 trial. J Hepatol 2012;56:S478–9.

15. Lok AS, Gardiner DF, Lawitz E, et al. Preliminary study of two antiviral agents for hepatitis C genotype 1. N Engl J Med 2012;366:216–24.

16. Lok AS, Gardiner DF, Hezode C, et al. Confirmation that quadruple therapy with daclatasvir (NS5A Inhibitor), asunaprevir (NS3 Inhibitor) and peginterferon/ribavirin results in high rate of SVR4 in HCV genotype 1 null responders. J Hepatol 2012;56(Suppl 2):S557.

17. Sulkowski MS, Gardiner DF, Lawitz F, et al. Potent viral suppression with all-oral combination of daclatasvir (NS5A inhibitor) and GS-7977 (NS5B inhibitor) +/- ribavirin, in treatment-naive patients with chronic HCV GT1, 2, or 3. J Hepatol 2012;56(Suppl 2):S560.

18. Chayama K, Takahashi S, Toyota J, et al. Dual therapy with the nonstructural protein 5A inhibitor, daclatasvir, and the nonstructural protein 3 protease inhibitor, asunaprevir, in hepatitis C virus genotype 1b-infected null responders. Hepatology 2012;55:742–8.

19. Suzuki F, Ikeda K, Toyota J, et al. Dual oral therapy with the NS5A inhibitor daclatasvir (BMS-790052) and NS3 protease inhibitor asunaprevir (BMS-650032)

in HCV genotype 1B-infected null responders or ineligible/intolerant to peginterferon/ribavirin. J Hepatol 2012;56(Suppl 2):S7–8.

20. Yang G, Wiles J, Patel D, et al. Preclinical characteristics of ACH-3102: a novel HCV NS5A inhibitor with improved potency against genotype-1A virus and variants resistant to 1st generation of NS5A inhibitors. J Hepatol 2012; 56(Suppl 2):S330.

21. Liu R, Kong R, Mann P, et al. In vitro resistance analysis of HCV NS5A inhibitor: MK-8742 demonstrates increased potency against clinical resistance variants and higher resistance barrier. J Hepatol 2012;56(Suppl 2):S334–5.

Non-nucleoside Analogue Polymerase Inhibitors in Development

Paul J. Pockros, MD

KEYWORDS

- Non-nucleoside analogue polymerase inhibitors (NNPI) • Hepatitis C • ABT-333
- B120712 • Filibuvir • Tegobuvir • Setrobuvir (ANA-598) • VX-222

KEY POINTS

- Four different allosteric binding sites have been identified for inhibition of the NS5B polymerase by non-nucleoside inhibitors (NNPIs).
- NNPIs display a low to medium antiviral activity and have a low genetic barrier to resistance, evidenced by frequent viral breakthrough in monotherapy studies and selection of resistance mutations at variable sites of the enzyme.
- In contrast to nucleoside analogues, NNPIs in general do not display antiviral activity against different hepatitis C virus genotypes.
- Because of their low antiviral efficacy and low genetic barrier to resistance, NNPIs will not be developed as part of triple therapy but rather as components of quadruple or all-oral regimens.
- Several drugs show genotype potency 1b >1a and/or IL28B genotype CC > non-CC benefit.
- Hyperbilirubinemia occurs with 2 of the drugs (tegobuvir and BI-207127).

INTRODUCTION

Four different allosteric binding sites have been identified for inhibition of the NS5B polymerase by non-nucleoside inhibitors (NNPIs). Currently, several non-nucleoside inhibitors are in phase I and II clinical evaluation, but only two have reached phase III development (**Table 1**).[1–3] **Fig. 1** shows the 4 different domains that current compounds have been designed to inhibit (Thumb domains 1 and 2, and Palm domains 1 and 2). Examples of drugs in development that inhibit each of these domains are discussed in more detail in this article.

Division of Gastroenterology/Hepatology, Scripps Clinic, 10666 North Torrey Pines Road, La Jolla, CA 92037, USA
E-mail address: pockros.paul@scrippshealth.org

Clin Liver Dis 17 (2013) 123–128
http://dx.doi.org/10.1016/j.cld.2012.09.004   liver.theclinics.com

Table 1
NS5B polymerase inhibitors

	Nucleos(t)ide Analogue	Non-nucleos(t)ide Inhibitors
Approved	None	None
Phase III	GS-7977	ABT-333, ABT-072
Phase II	NM283 (Idenix; development halted because of toxicity)	ANA-598
	R1626 (Roche: development halted because of toxicity)	B120712
	Mericitabine (R7128; Genentech/Roche)	Filibur
	PSI-938 (Pharmasett; development halted because of toxicity)	IDX-375
	INX-189 (Inhibitex/BMS; development halted because of toxicity)	Tegobuvir
	VX-135 (Alios/Vertex)	VCH-916
		VX-222

In general, these NNPIs display low to medium antiviral activity and have a low genetic barrier to resistance, evidenced by frequent viral breakthrough in monotherapy studies and selection of resistance mutations at variable sites of the enzyme (**Fig. 2**). For instance, a phase II triple therapy study with filibuvir plus pegylated interferon and ribavirin showed high relapse and relatively low sustained viral response (SVR) rates.[4] In contrast to nucleoside analogues, NNPIs in general do not display antiviral activity against different hepatitis C virus (HCV) genotypes.[5] Because of their low antiviral efficacy and low genetic barrier to resistance, NNPIs will not be developed as part of triple therapy but rather as components of quadruple or all-oral regimens with more potent drugs that have a higher barrier to resistance. Examples of such combinations currently in development are shown in **Box 1**.

NNPIS

The antiviral potency of NNPIs as monotherapy is less than that seen with NS3/4 protease inhibitors and is generally in the range of 0.5 and 3.5 (setrobuvir [ANA-598]).[5] Examples of the specific targets for NNPIs are Thumb domain 1 (BI-207127), Thumb domain 2 (filibuvir, VX-222), Palm domain 1 (setrobuvir [ANA-59], ABT-333,

HCV RNA Polymerase
Nucleoside and Non-nucleoside Inhibition

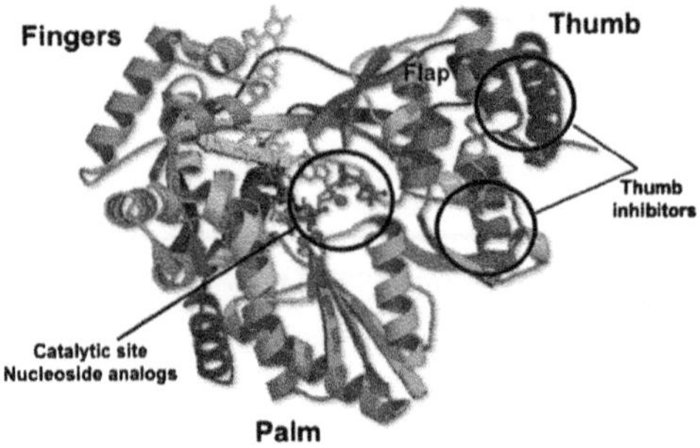

Fig. 1. The 4 different domains that current compounds have been designed to inhibit.

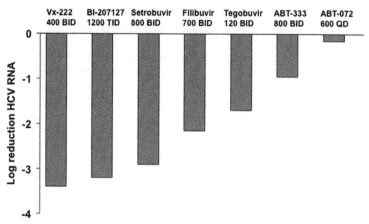

Fig. 2. The antiviral potency of non-nucleoside inhibitors as monotherapy. BID, twice daily; QD, daily; TID, 3 times a day.

ABT-072]), and Palm domain 2 (tegobuvir).[6–11] The efficacy, barrier to resistance, and adverse event data reported thus far in phase I and II trials is discussed in detail herein. In addition, results of the studies on interferon (IFN)-free combinations using these compounds are reviewed where data are available.

BI-207127 is an NNPI with potency as monotherapy of 3.2 $\log_{10}$ currently in phase II development. It has been tested together with pegylated interferon (PEG-IFN) and ribavirin (RBV) and shown to be relatively well tolerated except for the development of hyperbilirubinemia caused by hepatic transport enzyme inhibition.[8] BI-207127 has been studied in an all-oral combination with BI-201335, an NS3/4 protease inhibitor, and RBV.[8] In this study, treatment-naive genotype 1 (G1) patients received either 400 mg or 600 mg of BI-207127 3 times a day in combination with 120 mg of BI-201335 and weight-based RBV daily for 1 month; all patients then received BI-201335 and PEG-IFN + RBV until week 24. All the patients on the 600-mg dose had HCV RNA <25 IU/mL by week 3 of the triple drug regimen. Patients with G1a who received the 400-mg dose had viral relapses not seen with the 600-mg dose, suggesting that a subtype effect could be overcome with drug dosage. There were no viral relapses in patients with G1b at either dose.

This study was followed then by SOUND-C2 using BI 201335 at 120 mg daily + BI 207127 at 600 mg twice a day or 3 times a day ± weight-based RBV in treatment-naive G1 patients for either 16, 28, or 40 weeks.[12] This was a large randomized trial with

---

Box 1
Some interferon-free regimens in development using combinations with NNPIs

ABT-450/ritonavir + ABT-072 + ribavirin (RBV)[6]

ABT-450/ritonavir + ABT-333 + RBV[7]

BI-201335 + BI-207127 ± RBV[8]

Mericitabine + danoprevir/ritonavir + setrobuvir (ANA598-505) + RBV[9]

GS-9256 + tegobuvir (GS-9190) ± RBV[10]

GS-5885 + GS-9451 + tegobuvir + RBV[11]

a total of 362 patients and was the first data presented on an IFN-free regimen which included patients with cirrhosis. The results showed >80% SVR rates in all G1b and G1a patients who were IL28B CC allele. Patients who were G1a with CT or TT alleles had an SVR of 32%. The twice daily schedule seemed to perform as well as the 3 times a day schedule and would be preferable. The viral breakthroughs seen in the G1a patients suggest that the NNPI is not able to overcome the lower barrier of resistance to the protease inhibitor seen with this genotype. Unfortunately, this is a common theme with other drug combinations.

Filibuvir (FLV) is a moderately potent NNPI with a low barrier to resistance and has been studied in combination with PEG-IFN + RBV[4] but not in an IFN-free regimen. The IFN combination study evaluated treatment-naive, HCV G1 patients, who were randomized to receive FLV (200, 300, or 500 mg twice daily) or placebo (PBO) plus PEG-IFN (180 μg/wk) and RBV (1000/1200 mg/d) for 4 weeks, followed by open-label PEG-IFN/RBV from week 5 to week 48. The addition of FLV to PEG-IFN/RBV was well tolerated and markedly increased the rates of rapid virologic response (RVR) and complete early virologic response (cEVR). However, there were high relapse rates that may reflect the short duration of FLV administration, and the overall SVR rates were no better than placebo.

VX-222 is a relatively potent NNPI ($3.4 \log_{10}$ HCV RNA reduction) that has been studied in different combinations with telaprevir (TVR), PEG-IFN, and RBV. In the ZENITH study, the safety and efficacy of 2 dose levels of VX-222 100 or 400 mg twice daily with TVR 1125 mg twice daily either alone (DUAL), with RBV (TRIPLE), or with PEG-IFN/RBV (QUAD) in chronic HCV G1 treatment-naive patients.[13] Data suggest the DUAL arm was ineffective in all patients, while the TRIPLE arm was effective in a few G1a and all G1b patients. However most G1a patients had viral breakthroughs while on therapy and the number of G1b patients in the study was limited. The QUAD arm showed high SVR12 rates at doses of 100 mg and 400 mg of VX-222 (85% and 90%, respectively).

Setrobuvir (ANA-598) is an NNPI with reasonable potency as monotherapy ($-2.9 \log_{10}$) and has been studied in 2 separate phase II trials with PEG-IFN + RBV. In 1 of these studies, the drug was given at 200 mg or 400 mg twice daily with PEG-IFN + RBV for 12 weeks followed by PEG-IFN + RBV in a response-guided treatment regimen.[14] The triple combination arms demonstrated better RVR and early cRVR rates than the PEG-IFN + RBV arm, however there was no difference in SVR rates due to high rates of relapse. The drug seemed to be well tolerated. In a second phase IIb study, patients were administered 200 mg twice daily in combination therapy with PEG-IFN + RBV for 24 or 48 weeks to treatment-naive and treatment-experienced patients. Only interim safety data have been released from this study indicating that the adverse event profile is similar for the setrobuvir group and the control group; no formal data have been presented or published. Setrobuvir is currently in a combination trial using mericitabine + danoprevir/ritonavir + RBV.[9]

Two relatively weak NNPIs have each been tested separately in combination with a boosted potent protease inhibitor by Abbott Laboratories and shown very interesting data.[6,7] In the first, ABT-333, with a potency as monotherapy of only $-0.95 \log_{10}$ HCV RNA reduction, was given to treatment-naive or treatment-experienced G1 patients at 400 mg twice daily in combination with ABT-450/ritonavir 250/100 mg daily or ABT-450/ritonavir 150/100 mg daily and RBV. The treatment-naive patients showed remarkable SVR rates >90% at both doses of the regimens. However, the treatment-failure patients (who all received ABT-450/ritonavir 150/100 mg in a daily dose) showed SVR rates <50%.[7] A significant number of the patients in the study developed hyperbilirubinemia consistent with the known effect of ABT-450 on the OATP1B1 bilirubin transporter. There was also an effect on serum creatinine and creatinine clearance seen in 2 patients, which resolved without dose reduction. This combination regimen has moved into phase III development.

ABT-072 is the other NNPI from Abbott Laboratories tested in combination with the boosted protease inhibitor ABT-450. ABT-072 is only modestly potent as monotherapy (-1.57 $\log_{10}$ HCV RNA reduction) but also showed a remarkably high SVR rate when given in a single-arm, open-label, pilot study of ABT-450/r 150/100 mg daily + ABT-072 400 mg daily + weight-based RBV for 12 weeks (91%).[6] One patient in this small study developed late relapse at posttreatment week 36. The resistance variant observed in 99% of clones sequenced was to the NNPI compound (Y448H variant) rather than the protease inhibitor. It remains unclear if this is a one-time event or carries greater significance for these drug combinations.

Tegobuvir is an NNPI with reasonable potency as monotherapy (-1.7 $\log_{10}$ HCV RNA reduction) that has been tested with several other direct-acting antivirals in IFN-free combinations.[10,11] The initial study evaluated the combination with a protease inhibitor, GS-9256, 75 mg twice daily, and tegobuvir 40 mg twice daily with or without RBV. This 4-week study clearly demonstrated that viral breakthrough occurred rapidly if RBV was left out of the regimen.[10] A second study combined tegobuvir at 30 mg twice daily with a quadruple regimen of GS-5885 (NS5A inhibitor) and GS-9451 (protease inhibitor) with RBV. An interim analysis of the data from an ongoing study showed the 4-drug regimen provided high rates of SVR12 (81%) with 12-week therapy in noncirrhotic patients with G1. Virologic breakthrough and relapse rates were lower in G1b than G1a infection and virologic breakthrough was associated with the emergence of multidrug resistance. In addition, lower virologic breakthrough rates with IL28B CC versus non-CC genotype were seen. The regimen was well tolerated over 24 weeks of treatment.[11]

SUMMARY

NNPIs have several limitations including low to moderate potency, a low barrier to resistance, unlikely to cross genotype activity, genotype potency 1b >1a, and hyperbilirubinemia for 2 of the drugs (tegobuvir and BI-207127). These drugs will have no role in monotherapy and may have only a limited role in triple therapy with PEG-IFN + RBV. They could be part of a quadruple therapy regimen using PEG-IFN, RBV, PI/Nuc/NS5A plus non-nucleoside inhibitor or a triple or quadruple IFN-free regimen using a PI/Nuc/NS5A plus non-nucleoside inhibitor or a PI/ritonavir plus NPI plus non-nucleoside inhibitor plus RBV. Several issues remain unclear at the time of this review; the role of these compounds, including minimal dosing required, safety, and cost, remains to be clarified.

REFERENCES

1. Ali S, Leveque V, Le Pogam S, et al. Selected replicon variants with low-level in vitro resistance to the hepatitis C virus NS5B polymerase inhibitor PSI-6130 lack cross-resistance with R1479. Antimicrob Agents Chemother 2008;52:4356–69.
2. Cooper C, Lawitz E, Ghali P, et al. Antiviral activity of the non-nucleoside polymerase inhibitor, VCH-759, in chronic hepatitis C patients: results from a randomized, double-blind, placebo-controlled, ascending multiple dose study. Hepatology 2007;46: S864.
3. Erhardt A, Deterding K, Benhamou Y, et al. Safety, pharmacokinetics and antiviral effect of BILB 1941, a novel hepatitis C virus RNA polymerase inhibitor, after 5 days oral treatment. Antivir Ther 2009;14:23–32.

4. Jacobson I, Pockros P, Lalezari J, et al. Antiviral activity of filibuvir in combination with pegylated interferon alfa-2a and ribavirin for 28 days in treatment naïve patients chronically infected with HCV genotype 1. J Hepatol 2009;50(Suppl 1): S382.

5. Sarrazin C, Zeuzem S. Resistance to direct antiviral agents in patients with hepatitis C virus infection. Gastroenterology 2010;138:447–62.

6. Lawitz E, Poordad F, Kowdley KV, et al. A 12-week interferon-free regimen of ABT-450/r, ABT-072, and ribavirin was well tolerated and achieved sustained virologic response [abstract no. 13]. Presented at the 47th Annual Meeting of the European Association for the Study of the Liver. Barcelona (Spain), April 18–22, 2012.

7. Poordad F, Lawitz E, Kowdley KV, et al. 12-Week interferon-free regimen of ABT-450/r + ABT-333 + ribavirin achieved SVR12 in more than 90% of treatment-naïve HCV non-responders [abstract no. 1399]. Presented at the 47th Annual Meeting of the European Association for the Study of the Liver. Barcelona (Spain), April 18–22, 2012.

8. Zeuzem S, Asselah T, Angus P, et al. Efficacy of the protease inhibitor BI 201335, polymerase inhibitor BI 207127, and ribavirin in patients with chronic HCV infection. Gastroenterology 2011;141(6):2047–55.

9. Hoffmann-La Roche. ANNAPURNA: A study of the combination of RO5466731, RO5190591, ritonavir and Copegus (ribavirin) with or without RO5024048 in patients with chronic hepatitis C who are either treatment-naive or have previously experienced a null response to interferon-based treatment [ClinicalTrials.gov identifier NCT01628094]. US National Institutes of Health, ClinicalTrials.gov [online]. Available at: http://www.clinicaltrials.gov. Accessed August 26, 2012.

10. Zeuzem S, Buggisch P, Agarwal K, et al. Dual, triple, and quadruple combination treatment with a protease inhibitor (GS-9256) and a polymerase inhibitor (GS-9190) alone and in combination with ribavirin (RBV) or PEGIFN/RBV for up to 28 days in treatment-naive, genotype 1 HCV subjects [abstract no. LB1]. Presented at the 61st Annual Meeting of the American Association for the Study of Liver Diseases. Boston (MA), October 29–November 2, 2010.

11. Sulkowski M, Rodriguez-Torres M, Lawitz E, et al. High sustained virologic response rate in treatment-naive HCV genotype 1a and 1b patients treated for 12 weeks with an interferon-free all-oral quad regimen: interim results [abstract no. 1421]. Presented at the 47th Annual Meeting of the European Association for the Study of the Liver. Barcelona (Spain), April 18–22, 2012.

12. Zeuzem S, Soriano V, Asselah T, et al. SVR4 and SVR12 with an interferon-free regimen of BI201335 and BI207127, +/- ribavirin, in treatment-naïve patients with genotype-1 HCV infection: interim results of SOUND-C2 [abstract no. 101]. Presented at the 47th Annual Meeting of the European Association for the Study of the Liver. Barcelona (Spain), April 18–22, 2012.

13. Nelson DR, Gane EJ, Jacobson IM, et al. VX- 222/telaprevir in combination with peginterferon-alfa-2a and ribavirin in treatment-naive genotype 1 HCV patients treated for12 weeks: Zenith study, SVR 12 interim analyses [abstract]. Hepatology 2011;54:1442.

14. Lawitz E, Rodriguez-Torres M, Rustgi VK, et al. Safety and antiviral activity of ANA598 in combination with pegylated interferon α2A plus ribavirin in treatment-naïve genotype-1 chronic HCV patients [abstract no. LB13]. Presented at the 45th Annual Meeting of the European Association for the Study of the Liver (EASL 2010). Vienna (Austria), April 14–18, 2010.

Cyclophilin Inhibitors for Hepatitis C Therapy

Fernando E. Membreno, MD, MSc[a],*, Jennifer C. Espinales[b],
Eric J. Lawitz, MD, AGAF, CPI[a]

KEYWORDS

- Cyclophilin • Cyclophilin inhibitors • Debio 025 • NIM 811 • SCY-635 • Alisporivir
- Non-interferon • Interferon-free

KEY POINTS

- Cyclophilin inhibitors are effective at achieving a sustained viral response across all major Hepatitis C genotypes.
- Cyclophilin inhibitors are host targeted agents against Hepatitis C virus that have a pangenotypic spectrum and a high barrier to resistance.
- Cyclophilin inhibitors are capable of achieving a sustained virological response without the need of pegylated interferon, particularly in genotypes 2 and 3.

INTRODUCTION

The treatment of Hepatitis C (HCV) is rapidly changing with the advent of new combinations of direct-acting antivirals (DAAs) that are currently at different stages of clinical research development. In 2011, scientists and physicians, working intensively in this field, were rewarded with the approval of 2 first-generation protease inhibitors, Boceprevir[1,2] and Telaprevir,[3–6] to be used in conjunction with pegylated interferon (PEG-IFN) and Ribavirin (RBV). These new standard-of-care regimens led to an overall improvement in sustained virological response (SVR) in both naive and non-responder HCV patient populations, but unfortunately added even more challenges to an already difficult HCV therapy. After using these 2 regimens in clinical practice since their approval, the authors have encountered that patients have now been challenged with more pronounced side effects, anemia,[7,8] rash,[9] more medication interactions, enrichment of resistant viral variants, and more compliance difficulties because of the large amount and frequency of daily pills that need to be ingested. In addition,

[a] Alamo Medical Research, 621 Camden Street, Suite 202, San Antonio, TX 78215, USA;
[b] University of Texas at Brownsville, Department of Biological Sciences, 80 Fort Brown Street, Brownsville, TX 78520, USA
* Corresponding author. 621 Camden Street, Suite 202, San Antonio, TX 78215.
E-mail address: membreno@alamomedicalresearch.com

Clin Liver Dis 17 (2013) 129–139
http://dx.doi.org/10.1016/j.cld.2012.09.008
1089-3261/13/$ – see front matter © 2013 Elsevier Inc. All rights reserved.

patients who have been prioritized for these therapies are those with advanced liver fibrosis, who unfortunately are the ones who are prone to suffer more side effects, such as profound anemia and other cytopenias. These complications are difficult to control, requiring aggressive dose reductions of RBV and PEG-IFN or consideration for the use of growth factors.[10] As a result of all these difficulties with the current standard of care, the medical community continues to search for a simpler, less toxic, and more effective therapy that can cure more patients in a shorter period of time.

Cyclophilin inhibitors (CypI), because of their unique mechanism of action, pangenotypic spectrum, and low resistance rates, are now being considered a future HCV therapy that has shown exciting antiviral properties and the capacity to achieve an SVR, with and without IFN. In this review article, current thoughts on mechanism of action and the published studies that support the use of these Host Targeted Agents (HTAs) that have the possibility of becoming part of a new generation of HCV therapies in the future are presented.

MECHANISM OF ACTION OF CYCLOSPORIN A AND CYCLOPHILIN INHIBITORS

Cyclophilin A (CypA) is a host cellular protein that has a peptidyl-prolyl cis-trans isomerase activity that catalyzes the cis-trans isomerization of the prolyl peptide bond preceding proline residues.[11] CypA plays an important role in transmembrane transportation and viral replication, including human immunodeficiency virus (HIV) and HCV.[9,10,12–17] CypA, particularly, has been shown to be a crucial cofactor for HCV replication by interacting, directly or indirectly, with 3 nonstructural HCV proteins: NS5A, NS5B, and NS2.[11,18,19] Furthermore, there is evidence that CypA specifically binds to the NS5A protein domain II, catalyzing cis-trans isomerization, leading to inhibition of HCV replication.[20] Cyclophilin B (CypB) has been reported to enhance the activity of the HCV RNA polymerase (NS5B) by increasing the RNA-binding affinity.[21]

The first CypA inhibitor identified was the immunosuppressive drug Cyclosporine A (CSA), a compound originally isolated from the soil fungus *Tolypocladium inflatum*, that has shown clear evidence of anti-HCV activity both in vitro and in vivo.[22–29] Various point mutations in NS5A and NS5B have been associated with in vitro resistance to CSA.[30–33] Various studies have suggested that both NS5A and NS5B are ligands for CypA.[19,30–32,34,35] CSA has been shown to disrupt the interactions between NS5A with CypA-CypB and also NS5B with CypB.[36] Interestingly, a study showed that CypA binds to full-length NS5A from HCV genotypes 1a, 1b, 2a, and 2b that could contribute to the polygenotypic spectrum of CypA inhibitors. The same study demonstrated that CSA prevents the interaction between CypA and NS5A in a dose-dependent pattern.[34] Clinical studies in HCV treatment-naive patients receiving CSA for 24 weeks in combination with IFN have shown a rate of SVR of 55% (42/76) compared with IFN alone 31% (14/44), with the greatest benefit seen in genotype 1 high viral load patients. Side effects were similar among both groups.[27] A pilot study in 10 HCV nonresponders using a combination of alfacon-1 IFN with CSA (100 mg for 4 weeks and 50 mg for 44 weeks) showed that the rates of virologic response were disappointing.[37] Unfortunately, the immunosuppressive calcineurin inhibitor properties of CSA have limited its use in clinical practice.

There are now 3 nonimmunosuppressive Cyclophilin inhibitors that are undergoing clinical evaluation: Debio 025, NIM 811, and SCY-635. The mechanism of action of these molecules has been proposed to include the following: preventing cyclophilin A recruitment into the replication complex, interfering with NS5B polymerase activity, neutralizing NS5A activities, neutralizing NS2 activities, and inhibiting the assembly and release of viral particles.[19] Alisporivir (Debio 025) is a CypI derived from CSA, in phase 3 of clinical development. This molecule retains the binding affinity toward cyclophylins but does not inhibit calcineurin and therefore lacks the immunosuppressive properties of CSA.[38] Because these CypIs block host factors, they have a higher barrier for the development of resistance. A study with Alisporivir (ALV) demonstrated that it took an average of 20 weeks to select for resistant HCV replicons, compared with less than 2 weeks seen with protease inhibitors. Mutation D320E in the NS5A protein was the most consistently selected but conferred low-level resistance to ALV probably by reducing the need of CypA-dependent isomerization of NS5A. Importantly, there was no cross-resistance with NS3 protease and NS5B polymerase inhibitors.[11]

CYCLOPHYLIN INHIBITORS IN DEVELOPMENT
NIM811

NIM811, a nonimmunosuppressive cyclosporine analog, initially demonstrated potent antiviral properties that disrupt HIV replication and was also proved to exert anti-HCV properties in vitro at exceedingly lower concentrations than that of CSA.[39–41] A small alteration in NIM811, which is structurally comparable to cyclosporine except at position 4 whereby an isobutyl group is replaced by a sec-butyl group, essentially blocks the recognition site of CypA/cyclosporine by calcineurin and eradicates the immunosuppressive function linked with cyclosporine.[23] NIM811 efficiently reduced dose-dependent viral RNA in HCV replicon cells; however, with the combination of IFNα, it enhanced the anti-HCV activity without causing any increase in cytotoxicity.[23] Furthermore, combinations of NIM811 with HCV protease inhibitors (BILN2061) exerted additive properties, whereas with polymerase inhibitors, nucleoside (NM107), or a nonnucleoside (thiophene-2-carboxylic acid), exerted synergistic properties, leading to pronounced anti-HCV effects without causing any increase in cytotoxicity. Most notably, NIM811 was highly effective in blocking the emergence of resistance when used in combination with viral protease or polymerase inhibitors.[42] An initial dose-escalation study with 72 genotype 1 patients randomly assigned to 6 sequential cohorts receiving 25–600 mg every day or twice a day, assessed the safety, pharmacokinetic, and antiviral activity of NIM811. The compound was well tolerated, with no significant adverse effects except for mild, nonclinically significant elevations in bilirubin and decreased platelet counts in the 400-mg and 600-mg dosing groups.[43] NIM811 monotherapy showed an improvement in alanine aminotransferase levels, but no antiviral effect at doses between 25 mg every day and 600 mg twice a day.[44] In a phase 2, 14-day, randomized, double-blind, placebo-controlled trial, 21 HCV genotype 1 relapser patients received NIM811 in combination with PEG-IFN (n = 10) and 11 received PEG-IFN monotherapy. This study demonstrated that NIM811's antiviral effects were pronounced when combined with PEG-IFNα2a with a mean viral load reduction of -2.85 $\log_{10}$ in the combination therapy arms compared with -0.56 $\log_{10}$ with PEG-IFN monotherapy. ALT decreased significantly in the combination group compared with the PEG-IFN monotherapy arm. Liver transaminase normalization occurred at doses greater than 75 mg, suggesting a hepatocytoprotective effect of this compound. As in the prior study, there were no severe or serious adverse events, with the most common side effects being thrombocytopenia (mean platelets, 203×10^9/L at baseline; dropping to 105×10^9/L by day 14). The use of NIM811 was associated with an increase in bilirubin; however, this increase was not considered clinically significant.[45] Interestingly, several studies using NIM811 have shown a hepatoprotective effect and possibly antifibrotic features due to suppression of collagen production and increased collagenases activity.[46–48]

SCY-635

SCY-635, a nonimmunosuppressive CsA analog, is currently under phase 2 of clinical development. Preclinical studies have demonstrated that SCY-635 is a competitive, reversible inhibitor of the peptidyl prolyl isomerase activity expressed by CypA that exerts potent anti-HCV effects in vitro.[49] A proposed mechanism is that SCY-635 prevents CypA-NS5A interactions in a dose-dependent manner in genotypes 1 to 3.[50] By preventing the formation of these complexes, SCY-635 blocks viral replication.[50] Two-drug synergy studies indicate that SCY-635 exhibits additive to synergistic antiviral activity when tested in vitro with IFNα-2b or ribavirin without increasing cell cytotoxicity.[49,51] In addition to antiviral effects, SCY-635 also shows antifibrotic properties shown in in vitro HCV studies.[52]

A phase 1b study evaluated 20 adults with chronic HCV genotype 1. All patients enrolled were men and 75% of the patients were African American. They were randomized to SCY-635 oral doses of 100, 200, or 300 mg 3 times a day for 15 days. At 900 mg (300 mg 3 times a day), SCY-635 resulted in serum concentrations exceeding EC_{50}, and at day 15 it was reaching levels close to EC_{90} with concentrations of 463 ng/mL (350 nM). The most prominent HCV RNA decrease occurred in 2 subjects with IL28B genotype CC (viral load reduction of −2.34 and −5.47 $\log_{10}$ IU/mL), suggesting the potential mechanism of antiviral activity of SCY-635 linked with IFN. The mean HCV viral load reduction was −2.24 $\log_{10}$ IU/mL. A interesting observation was the parallel association between serum SCY-635 concentrations and plasma levels for all markers (IFNα, IFNλ1, IFNλ3, and 2′5′oligoadenylate synthetase 1 [2′5′OAS-1]), especially the concordance between the absorption and disposition of SCY-635 and changes in the plasma protein concentrations of endogenous IFNs and 2′5′OAS-1. Treatment with SCY-635 increased plasma protein concentrations in endogenous type I and III IFNs and dependent on stimulated genes, 2′5′OAS-1, suggesting that SCY-635 is involved in the restoration of the innate immune response against chronic HCV infection. However, plasma IFNβ concentrations were significantly reduced with the escalating serum concentrations of SCY-635. The specific suppression of IFNβ did not diminish the clinical antiviral activity of SCY-635. The treatment-associated increases in the plasma protein concentrations of IFNα, IFNλ1, and IFNλ3 imply that cyclophilins play opposing roles in regulating the production of IFNβ in comparison to IFNα, IFNλ1, and IFNλ3. The most common side effects were headache, nausea, and transient elevations of serum creatinine phosphokinase and liver function tests. One patient experienced a severe single elevation in serum triglycerides, possibly treatment-related, that was modified by proper diet.[53]

In vitro studies indicate that resistance to SCY-635 requires multiple mutations in the NS5A and NS5B replication complex proteins.[54] Clinical studies have been consistent with these results, by demonstrating that the administration of 900 mg SCY-635 as monotherapy is sufficient to establish a high genetic barrier for the selection of resistant HCV variants with no evidence of mutations in NS5A and with minimal evidence of resistance selection in NS5B.[55] A phase 2a study was recently completed on HCV-naive, genotype 1, IL-28B non-CC patients. The study design involved the addition of SCY-635 to PEG-IFN/RBV therapy for 4 weeks followed by continuation of PEG-IFN/RBV for an additional 24 weeks. Results have yet to be released.[56]

Alisporivir

Alisporivir (Debio-025), an analog of cyclosporine A, is a host-targeting antiviral cyclophilin inhibitor currently in phase III clinical trials. It demonstrates a stronger Cyp binding and ×10 higher antiviral effects caused by changes in position 3 and low immunosuppressive activity (no calcineurin binding) caused by changes in position 4 of the Debio-025 molecule.[18,57]

In preclinical studies, ALV demonstrated to prevent/delay resistance development against the protease inhibitors Telaprevir and BILN-2601 and the polymerase inhibitors RI479 and JT-16, even at concentrations as low as 0.1 μM.[58] The only significant mutation related to ALV is D32OE, but its presence is not sufficient to cause a viral breakthrough.[11]

In a phase 1 study using ALV in asymptomatic HIV-1–monoinfected and HIV-1/HCV–coinfected patients, ALV showed a mean HCV RNA reduction of $-3.6 \log_{10}$ after 14 days with oral treatment of 2400 mg daily. Patients with genotype 3 achieved a maximum HCV RNA reduction of $-4.46 \log_{10}$ compared with a reduction of $-3.19 \log_{10}$ in patients with genotype 1 and 4. ALV showed the absence of viral breakthrough during treatment, which indicates that ALV has a high barrier for the selection of resistance.[59]

In a phase IIa study the combination of ALV and PEG-IFNα2a was investigated in treatment-naive HCV patients using escalating doses of ALV 200, 600, 1000 mg twice a day for week 1 and once a day for the following 3 weeks, in treatment-naive HCV patients compared with a placebo combined with PEG-IFNα2a. At week 4, patients with genotypes 1 and 4 who were given the 600-mg and 1000-mg combination treatment had HCV RNA reductions of -4.61 ± 1.88 and $-4.75 \pm 2.19 \log_{10}$ IU/mL, respectively. Patients with genotypes 2 and 3, at week 1, showed an HCV RNA reduction of -4.29 ± 1.03 and $-4.48 \pm 0.68 \log_{10}$ IU/mL, respectively, and at week 4, a reduction of -5.91 ± 1.11 and $-5.89 \pm 0.43 \log_{10}$ IU/mL, respectively. By day 22, most of the patients achieved undetectable HCV RNA and the addition of ALV was shown to increase the proportion of patients achieving a Rapid Virological Response (RVR). The results of this study showed that ALV has a potent activity against the 4 most prevalent HCV genotypes in treatment-naive patients, which is an attractive property of ALV not present in the first-generation DAA.[60]

A phase IIb study investigated triple therapy with ALV, PEG-IFNα2a, and RBV compared with PEG-IFNα2a and RBV alone. The study included 288 treatment-naive, genotype 1 HCV patients treated for 48 weeks. One arm of the study used response-guided therapy either for 24 or 48 weeks of ALV. ALV-based triple therapy for 24 weeks produced a rate of SVR of 53% that was similar to the rate of SVR of 55% in the control arm treated with 48 weeks of PEG-IFNα2a + RBV. ALV triple therapy for 48 weeks had rates of SVR as high as 76% compared with 55% in the PEG-IFNα2a and RBV control arm. This high rate of SVR with ALV triple therapy was achieved even with a low prevalence rate (19%) of IL28B-CC allele compared with that in the PEG-IFNα2a and RBV arm (33%). However, the most significant improvement was an SVR rate of 73% in patients with the IL28B-TT allele compared with an SVR rate of 17% in the control arm, and 100% rate of SVR in patients with the CC allele when treated with the ALV triple therapy for 48 weeks. Patients with undetectable HCV RNA at week 4 in the ALV triple therapy arm group were 3 times more likely to achieve an SVR than those treated with PEG-IFNα2a and RBV. A higher number of HCV null responders, defined as those achieving less than a 2 log drop in HCV RNA at week 12, were observed in the group receiving PEG-IFNα2a and RBV alone (9.6%), compared with those arms receiving ALV (0%). Also, the rate of relapse in ALV treatment (16%) was lower than in controls (24%). This trial demonstrated that an ALV-containing regimen is comparable to the efficacy of the first-generation protease inhibitors.[61]

A study by Nelson and colleagues[62] on HCV null nonresponders evaluated the efficacy and safety of ALV in 50 HCV, genotype 1 patients. The study consisted of 6 arms with various ALV doses (400–800 mg daily) in combination with PEG-IFN and RBV and an arm with an initial loading dose (400 mg twice a day for 7 days). The results demonstrated that ALV 400 mg daily monotherapy did not show any antiviral activity. The best antiviral response was obtained with ALV 400 mg daily (with initial loading dose) and ALV 800 mg daily for 29 days, showing a significant reduction in HCVRNA of $-1.96 \pm 1.25 \log_{10}$ and $-2.38 \pm 1.44 \log_{10}$ IU/mL, respectively. Three of 50 patients developed a reversible increase in bilirubin greater than 3 mg/dL (range 3.1–4.5).

The FUNDAMENTAL study evaluated the use of ALV triple therapy (ALV/PEG-IFN/RBV) in 461 HCV genotype 1 nonresponders (51%) and relapsers (43%), stratified by IL28B genotype, randomized into 4 treatment arms (ALV 600 mg qd, n = 121; ALV 800 mg qd, n = 117; ALV 400 mg bid, n = 109; and PR, n = 114). Compensated cirrhosis was present in 24% of patients. Complete EVR data have been reported, showing that ALV 400 mg twice a day with PEG-IFN/RBV was the most efficacious dose, achieving complete EVR in 73% relapsers, 70% null nonresponders, and 68% partial nonresponders. This study arm (ALV 400 mg twice a day) also had a higher frequency of side effects (hyperbilirubinemia [19%], thrombocytopenia [14%], neutropenia [32%], nausea [43%] compared with PEG-IFN/RBV). According to the authors, the treatment has been well tolerated and rates of discontinuation have been low and similar across all study arms. Although the study is ongoing, the data thus far are promising as a future therapeutic alternative for difficult-to-treat HCV populations.[63]

Another phase IIb study (VITAL-1) was performed to evaluate the combination of ALV $\pm$ RBV without PEG-IFNα. A total of 334 treatment-naive patients, genotype 2 and 3, were randomly assigned to receive the following: ALV, 1000 mg daily (n = 82); ALV, 800 mg daily and RBV (n = 94); ALV, 600 mg daily and RBV (n = 84); ALV, 600 mg daily and PEG-IFN (n = 39); versus a control arm of PEG-IFN and Ribavirin (n = 35). About 40% of patients achieved an RVR, and 97% of them remained HCV RNA negative by week 12. About 28% of patients who received ALV monotherapy achieved RVR and 91% of them remained HCV RNA negative by week 12. The remaining patients who did not achieve an RVR received triple therapy (ALV + PEG-IFNα2a + RBV) starting from week 6; this triple therapy allowed them to achieve an increase in their rate of response between 92% and 100% at week 12.[64] Recent data presented at EASL 2012 showed that patients who achieved an RVR and were kept on the IFN-free arms achieved an SVR12 between 82% and 93%. As expected, patients in the IFN-free arms had a lower rate of side effects compared with the other IFN-containing arms; however, a significant incidence of hyperbilirubinemia was observed during clinical trials.[65] ALV-induced hyperbilirubinemia is caused by the 3 following factors: (1) indirect increase in bilirubin is seen because of impairment in the OATP transporters of bilirubin into the hepatocytes; (2) direct hyperbilirubinemia is a consequence of impairment in the MRP2 excretion transporters of bilirubin within the hepatocytes; and (3) RBV-related hemolysis is seen. Most importantly, in clinical trials, ALT activity normalized faster in the ALV arms than in the non-ALV control arms and did not correlate with hyperbilirubinemia.[15] In this study ALV demonstrated to be effective in genotypes 2 or 3, even without the use of PEG-IFN.

ALV has demonstrated good tolerance and discontinuation because serious adverse effects have been relatively low. Frequency of clinical and laboratory adverse effects, except for hyperbilirubinemia, was similar across all the studied arms and comparable to controls receiving PEG-IFNα2a and RBV. Among 639 patients who received ALV in phase II studies, only 16 (2.5%) demonstrated a significant hyperbilirubinemia (exceeding levels 5$\times$ above norm). ALT activity normalized faster in arms containing ALV than controls treated without ALV.[60–62,64] ALV has attractive attributes that include its pangenotypic activity, once daily dosing (because of its calculated half-life of 60–90 hours[59]), and good safety profile. These promising results led to a phase III program that was ongoing as of April 2012; however, at that time the US Food and Drug Administration placed the ALV program on a full clinical hold and consequently all ALV-treated patients had to discontinue therapy. This clinical hold was due to a cluster of 3 cases of acute pancreatitis, one of them fatal, in the treatment group receiving ALV-based triple therapy.[66,67]

SUMMARY

The current therapy for HCV has improved dramatically since the use of IFN monotherapy in the early 1990s. Now, with the advent of protease inhibitors, overall rates of SVR of about 75% in patients with HCV genotype 1 have been achieved; unfortunately, a more complex therapy with additional adverse events has also been gained. Actually, at this point, it is uncertain whether the completion rates of triple therapy (PEG-IFN-RBV-Protease Inhibitor [Telaprevir or Boceprevir]) will mirror the rates seen in registered clinical trials. It is our impression that because of the selection of patients with advanced liver disease, prior nonresponders, comorbidities that were excluded from clinical trials (psychiatric diseases, immunologic, renal failure, obesity, etc), various medication interactions, and compliance issues, more patients may be unable to complete therapy. Agents such as CypI will be important additions to the HCV treatment paradigm if they are able to simplify and shorten therapy. ALV development is likely to move forward, but will not be used in conjunction with PEG-IFN because of a potential risk of acute pancreatitis. Certainly, this is only the beginning, and data of ALV in non-IFN phase 2 study arms have been very encouraging in genotype 2 and 3 patients. The mechanism of action of these CypIs is unique, affecting host instead of viral proteins, conferring them a high barrier to viral resistance. Furthermore, ALV has the potential to be a cornerstone agent for an IFN-free regimen when combined with DAAs, because it has a high barrier to resistance, no cross-resistance with other DAAs, and a pangenotypic spectrum. Few DAAs in development have the properties of a cornerstone agent; thus, further data in the use of ALV in an IFN-free treatment paradigm is welcomed.

REFERENCES

1. Poordad F, McCone J Jr, Bacon BR, et al. Boceprevir for untreated chronic HCV genotype 1 infection. N Engl J Med 2011;364(13):1195–206.
2. Kwo PY, Lawitz EJ, McCone J, et al. Efficacy of boceprevir, an NS3 protease inhibitor, in combination with peginterferon alfa-2b and ribavirin in treatment-naive patients with genotype 1 hepatitis C infection (SPRINT-1): an open-label, randomised, multicentre phase 2 trial. Lancet 2010;376(9742):705–16.
3. Hezode C, Forestier N, Dusheiko G, et al. Telaprevir and peginterferon with or without ribavirin for chronic HCV infection. N Engl J Med 2009;360(18):1839–50.
4. Jacobson IM, McHutchison JG, Dusheiko G, et al. Telaprevir for previously untreated chronic hepatitis C virus infection. N Engl J Med 2011;364(25):2405–16.
5. McHutchison JG, Everson GT, Gordon SC, et al. Telaprevir with peginterferon and ribavirin for chronic HCV genotype 1 infection. N Engl J Med 2009;360(18):1827–38.
6. Zeuzem S, Andreone P, Pol S, et al. Telaprevir for retreatment of HCV infection. N Engl J Med 2011;364(25):2417–28.

7. Poordad F, Lawitz E, Reddy K, et al. A Randomized Trial comparing ribavirin dose reduction versus erythropoietin for anemia management in previously untreated patients with chronic hepatitis C receiving boceprevir plus pginterferon/riba. 47th International Liver Congress (EASL 2012). [abstract: 1419]. Barcelona, April 18–22, 2012.

8. Sulkowski M, Roberts S, Afdhal N, et al. Ribavirin dose modification in treatment-naive and previously treated patients who received telaprevir combination treatment: no impact on sustained virologic response in phase 3 studies. 47th International Liver Congress (EASL 2012). [abstract: 1162]. Barcelona, April 18–22, 2012.

9. Hezode C. Boceprevir and telaprevir for the treatment of chronic hepatitis C: safety management in clinical practice. Liver Int 2012;32(Suppl 1):32–8.

10. Ghany MG, Nelson DR, Strader DB, et al. An update on treatment of genotype 1 chronic hepatitis C virus infection: 2011 practice guideline by the American Association for the Study of Liver Diseases. Hepatology 2011;54(4):1433–44.

11. Coelmont L, Hanoulle X, Chatterji U, et al. DEB025 (Alisporivir) inhibits hepatitis C virus replication by preventing a cyclophilin A induced cis-trans isomerisation in domain II of NS5A. PLoS One 2010;5(10):e13687.

12. Fischer G, Wittmann-Liebold B, Lang K, et al. Cyclophilin and peptidyl-prolyl cis-trans isomerase are probably identical proteins. Nature 1989;337(6206): 476–8.

13. Yang F, Robotham JM, Nelson HB, et al. Cyclophilin A is an essential cofactor for hepatitis C virus infection and the principal mediator of cyclosporine resistance in vitro. J Virol 2008;82(11):5269–78.

14. Gothel SF, Marahiel MA. Peptidyl-prolyl cis-trans isomerases, a superfamily of ubiquitous folding catalysts. Cell Mol Life Sci 1999;55(3):423–36.

15. Flisiak R, Parfieniuk-Kowerda A. Cyclophilin inhibitors. Curr Hepat Rep 2012; 11(3):153–9.

16. Ylinen LM, Schaller T. Cyclophilin A levels dictate infection efficiency of human immunodeficiency virus type 1 capsid escape mutants A92E and G94D. J Virol 2009;83(4):2044–7.

17. Strebel K, Luban J, Jeang KT. Human cellular restriction factors that target HIV-1 replication. BMC Med 2009;7:48.

18. Gallay PA. Cyclophilin inhibitors. Clin Liver Dis 2009;13(3):403–17.

19. Fischer G, Gallay P, Hopkins S. Cyclophilin inhibitors for the treatment of HCV infection. Curr Opin Investig Drugs 2010;11(8):911–8.

20. Foster TL, Gallay P, Stonehouse NJ, et al. Cyclophilin A interacts with domain II of hepatitis C virus NS5A and stimulates RNA binding in an isomerase-dependent manner. J Virol 2011;85(14):7460–4.

21. Watashi K, Ishii N, Hijikata M, et al. Cyclophilin B is a functional regulator of hepatitis C virus RNA polymerase. Mol Cell 2005;19(1):111–22.

22. Ishii N, Watashi K, Hishiki T, et al. Diverse effects of cyclosporine on hepatitis C virus strain replication. J Virol 2006;80(9):4510–20.

23. Ma S, Boerner JE, TiongYip C, et al. NIM811, a cyclophilin inhibitor, exhibits potent in vitro activity against hepatitis C virus alone or in combination with alpha interferon. Antimicrob Agents Chemother 2006;50(9):2976–82.

24. Nakagawa M, Sakamoto N, Enomoto N, et al. Specific inhibition of hepatitis C virus replication by cyclosporin A. Biochem Biophys Res Commun 2004;313(1): 42–7.

25. Watashi K, Hijikata M, Hosaka M, et al. Cyclosporin A suppresses replication of hepatitis C virus genome in cultured hepatocytes. Hepatology 2003;38(5):1282–8.

26. Akiyama H, Yoshinaga H, Tanaka T, et al. Effects of cyclosporin A on hepatitis C virus infection in bone marrow transplant patients. Bone marrow transplantation team. Bone Marrow Transplant 1997;20(11):993–5.

27. Inoue K, Sekiyama K, Yamada M, et al. Combined interferon alpha2b and cyclosporin A in the treatment of chronic hepatitis C: controlled trial. J Gastroenterol 2003;38(6):567–72.

28. Inoue K, Yoshiba M. Interferon combined with cyclosporine treatment as an effective countermeasure against hepatitis C virus recurrence in liver transplant patients with end-stage hepatitis C virus related disease. Transplant Proc 2005; 37(2):1233–4.

29. Tang H. Cyclophilin inhibitors as a novel HCV therapy. Viruses 2010;2:1621–34.

30. Fernandes F, Poole DS, Hoover S, et al. Sensitivity of hepatitis C virus to cyclosporine A depends on nonstructural proteins NS5A and NS5B. Hepatology 2007;46(4):1026–33.

31. Goto K, Watashi K, Inoue D, et al. Identification of cellular and viral factors related to anti-hepatitis C virus activity of cyclophilin inhibitor. Cancer Sci 2009;100(10): 1943–50.

32. Puyang X, Poulin DL, Mathy JE, et al. Mechanism of resistance of hepatitis C virus replicons to structurally distinct cyclophilin inhibitors. Antimicrob Agents Chemother 2010;54(5):1981–7.

33. Robida JM, Nelson HB, Liu Z, et al. Characterization of hepatitis C virus subgenomic replicon resistance to cyclosporine in vitro. J Virol 2007;81(11): 5829–40.

34. Chatterji U, Lim P, Bobardt MD, et al. HCV resistance to cyclosporin A does not correlate with a resistance of the NS5A-cyclophilin A interaction to cyclophilin inhibitors. J Hepatol 2010;53(1):50–6.

35. Kaul A, Stauffer S, Berger C, et al. Essential role of cyclophilin A for hepatitis C virus replication and virus production and possible link to polyprotein cleavage kinetics. PLoS Pathog 2009;5(8):e1000546.

36. Fernandes F, Ansari IU, Striker R. Cyclosporine inhibits a direct interaction between cyclophilins and hepatitis C NS5A. PLoS One 2010;5(3):e9815.

37. Cotler SJ, Morrissey MJ, Wiley TE, et al. A pilot study of the combination of cyclosporin A and interferon alfacon-1 for the treatment of hepatitis C in previous nonresponder patients. J Clin Gastroenterol 2003;36(4):352–5.

38. Landrieu I, Hanoulle X, Bonachera F, et al. Structural basis for the nonimmunosuppressive character of the cyclosporin A analogue Debio 025. Biochemistry 2010;49(22):4679–86.

39. Billich A, Hammerschmid F, Peichl P, et al. Mode of action of SDZ NIM 811, a nonimmunosuppressive cyclosporin A analog with activity against human immunodeficiency virus (HIV) type 1: interference with HIV protein-cyclophilin A interactions. J Virol 1995;69(4):2451–61.

40. Rosenwirth B, Billich A, Datema R, et al. Inhibition of human immunodeficiency virus type 1 replication by SDZ NIM 811, a nonimmunosuppressive cyclosporine analog. Antimicrob Agents Chemother 1994;38(8):1763–72.

41. Goto K, Watashi K, Murata T, et al. Evaluation of the anti-hepatitis C virus effects of cyclophilin inhibitors, cyclosporin A, and NIM811. Biochem Biophys Res Commun 2006;343(3):879–84.

42. Mathy JE, Ma S, Compton T, et al. Combinations of cyclophilin inhibitor NIM811 with hepatitis C virus NS3-4A protease or NS5B polymerase inhibitors enhance antiviral activity and suppress the emergence of resistance. Antimicrob Agents Chemother 2008;52(9):3267–75.

43. KE J, Lawitz E, Rozier R, et al. Safety, and tolerability of NIM811, a novel cyclophilin inhibitor for HCV, following single and multiple ascending dose, in healthy volunteers and HCV-infected patients. J Hepatol 2009;50(Suppl 1):S229.

44. Lawitz E, Rouzier R, Nguyen T, et al. Safety and antiviral efficacy of 14 days of the cycophilin inhibitor NIM811 in combination with pegylated interferon a2A in relapsed genotype 1 HCV infected patients. Oral Presentation at EASL 44th Annual Meeting, April 22–26, 2009, Copenhagen, Denmark.

45. Lawitz E, Godofsky E, Rouzier R, et al. Safety, pharmacokinetics, and antiviral activity of the cyclophilin inhibitor NIM811 alone or in combination with pegylated interferon in HCV-infected patients receiving 14 days of therapy. Antiviral Res 2011;89(3):238–45.

46. Theruvath TP, Zhong Z, Pediaditakis P, et al. Minocycline and N-methyl-4-isoleucine cyclosporin (NIM811) mitigate storage/reperfusion injury after rat liver transplantation through suppression of the mitochondrial permeability transition. Hepatology 2008;47(1):236–46.

47. Kohjima M, Enjoji M, Higuchi N, et al. NIM811, a nonimmunosuppressive cyclosporine analogue, suppresses collagen production and enhances collagenase activity in hepatic stellate cells. Liver Int 2007;27(9):1273–81.

48. Rehman H, Sun J, Shi Y, et al. NIM811 prevents mitochondrial dysfunction, attenuates liver injury, and stimulates liver regeneration after massive hepatectomy. Transplantation 2011;91(4):406–12.

49. Hopkins S, Scorneaux B, Huang Z, et al. SCY-625, a novel nonimmunosuppressive analog of cyclosporine that exhibits potent inhibition of hepatitis C virus RNA replication in vitro. Antimicrob Agents Chemother 2010;54(2):660–72.

50. Hopkins S, Bobardt M, Chatterji U, et al. The cyclophilin inhibitor SCY-635 disrupts HCV NS5A-Cyclophilin A complexes. Antimicrob Agents Chemother 2012;56(7):3888–97.

51. Hopkins S, Heuman D, Gavis E, et al. Safety, plasma, pharmacokinetics, and antiviral activity of SCY-635 in adult patients with chronic hepatitis C virus infection. J Hepatol 2009;50:S36.

52. Scorneaux B, Thomas G, Hopkins S, et al. The effects of SCY-635 a nonimmunosuppressive cyclosporin analog on stellate cell proliferation, collagen synthesis, TIMP-1 and collagenase production. J Hepatol 2010;52:S260.

53. Hopkins S, DiMassimo B, Rusnak P, et al. The cyclophilin inhibitor SCY-635 suppresses viral replication and induces endogenous interferons in patients with chronic HCV genotype 1 infection. J Hepatol 2012;57(1):47–54.

54. Hopkins S, Scorneaux B, Huang Z, et al. The genetic and biochemical basis for resistance to SCY-635. Hepatology 2008;48(S1):1019A–187A.

55. Hopkins S, Mosier S, Harris R, et al. 34 resistance selection following 15 days of monotherapy with SCY-635 a non-immunosuppressive cyclophilin inhibitor with potent anti-HCV activity. J Hepatol 2010;52:S15.

56. A phase 2a study of SCY-635 in combination with peginterferon Alfa-2a (Pegasys) and ribavirin (Copegus) in treatment-naive subjects with genotype 1 hepatitis C infection. Available at: Clinicaltrials.gov. Accessed July 25, 2012.

57. Hansson MJ, Mattiasson G, Mansson R, et al. The nonimmunosuppressive cyclosporin analogs NIM811 and UNIL025 display nanomolar potencies on permeability transition in brain-derived mitochondria. J Bioenerg Biomembr 2004;36:407–13.

58. Coelmont L, Paeshuyse J, Kaptein S, et al. The cyclophilin inhibitor Debio-025 is a potent inhibitor of hepatitis C virus replication in vitro with a unique resistance profile. Antiviral Res 2007;74(3):A39.

59. Flisiak R, Horban A, Gallay P, et al. The cyclophilin inhibitor Debio-025 shows potent anti-hepatitis C effect in patients coinfected with hepatitis C and human immunodeficiency virus. Hepatology 2008;47(3):817–26.
60. Flisiak R, Feinman SV, Jablkowski M, et al. The cyclophilin inhibitor Debio 025 combined with peg-IFNa2a significantly reduces viral load in treatment-naive hepatitis C patients. Hepatology 2009;49(5):1460–8.
61. Flisiak R, Pawlotsky JM, Crabbe R, et al. Once daily alisporivir (DEB025) plus pegifnalfa2a/ribavirin results in superior sustained virologic response (SVR24) in chronic hepatitis C genotype 1 treatment naive patients. J Hepatol 2011;54:S2.
62. Nelson DR, Ghalib RH, Sulkowski M, et al. Efficacy and safety of the cyclophilin inhibitor DEBIO 025 in combination with pegylated interferon alpha-2A and ribavirin in previously null-responder genotype 1 HCV patients. J Hepatol 2009;50:S40.
63. Alberti A, Chuang W, Flisiak R, et al. Alisporivir (ALV) plus PEG-interferon/ribavirin (PR) in HCV G1 treatment-experienced patients achieves primary endpoint with superior efficacy at treatment week 12 compared to retreatment with PR. J Hepatol 2012;54(Suppl 1):S2.
64. Pawlotsky JM, Flisiak R, Rasenack J, et al. Once daily alisporivir, interferon (IFN)-free regimens achieve high rates of early HCV clearance in previously untreated patients with HCV genotype (G) 2 or 3. Hepatology 2011;54(S1):1433A–55A.
65. Membreno F, Lawitz E. Non-interferon therapies for hepatitis C. Curr Hepat Rep 2012;11(3):146–52.
66. Alisporivir with pegIFN/RBV in protease inhibitor (PI) treatment failure patients with chronic hepatitis C. Available at: http://clinicaltrials.gov/ct2/show/NCT01500772?term=alisporivir&rank=1. Accessed July 25, 2012.
67. Novartis.com. Novartis Q1 2012 interim financial report—supplementary data. Available at: http://www.novartis.com/downloads/investors/financial-results/quarterly-results/q1-2012-interim-financial-report-en.pdf. Accessed July 25, 2012.

Index

Note: Page numbers of article titles are in **boldface** type.

Clin Liver Dis 17 (2013) 141–146
http://dx.doi.org/10.1016/S1089-3261(12)00135-3
1089-3261/13/$ – see front matter © 2013 Elsevier Inc. All rights reserved.

Moving?

Make sure your subscription moves with you!

To notify us of your new address, find your **Clinics Account Number** (located on your mailing label above your name), and contact customer service at:

Email: journalscustomerservice-usa@elsevier.com

800-654-2452 (subscribers in the U.S. & Canada)
314-447-8871 (subscribers outside of the U.S. & Canada)

Fax number: 314-447-8029

Elsevier Health Sciences Division
Subscription Customer Service
3251 Riverport Lane
Maryland Heights, MO 63043

*To ensure uninterrupted delivery of your subscription, please notify us at least 4 weeks in advance of move.

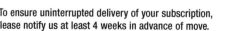

Printed and bound by CPI Group (UK) Ltd, Croydon, CR0 4YY

03/10/2024

01040436-0010